Copyright © 2019 Nina Brazer
All rights reserved.

Medical Disclaimer:

This book details the author's personal experiences and opinions about cancer. The author is not a [or your] healthcare provider. The author and publisher are providing this book and its contents on an "as is" basis and make no representations or warranties of any kind with respect to this book or its contents. The author and publisher disclaim all such representations and warranties, including for example warranties of merchantability and healthcare for a particular purpose. In addition, the author and publisher do not represent or warrant that the information accessible via this book is accurate, complete or current. The statements made about products and services have not been evaluated by the U.S. Food and Drug Administration. They are not intended to diagnose, treat, cure, or prevent any condition or disease. Please consult with your own physician or healthcare specialist regarding the suggestions and recommendations made in this book. Except as specifically stated in this book, neither the author or publisher, nor any authors, contributors, or other representatives will be liable for damages arising out of or in connection with the use of this book. This is a comprehensive limitation of liability that applies to all damages of any kind, including (without limitation) compensatory; direct, indirect or consequential damages; loss of data, income or profit; loss of or damage to property and claims of third parties. You understand that this book is not intended as a substitute for consultation with a licensed healthcare practitioner, such as your physician. Before you begin any healthcare program or change your lifestyle in any way, you will consult your physician or another licensed healthcare practitioner to ensure that you are in good health and that the examples contained in this book will not harm you. This book provides content related to physical and/or mental health issues. As such, the use of this book implies your acceptance of this disclaimer.

Table of contents

Forward	3
Why this Book Matters	8
My own journey with cancer	10
What I have learned on my journey and wish I knew before being diagnosed with cancer:	35
What is cancer?	35
The recurrence of cancer	40
Don't fear cancer	42
What is needed for a successful recovery?	44
Deal with the diagnosis	44
Deal with the battle in your own mind	46
Become a partner in the management of your recovery	48
Factors that influence a successful recovery	55
A holistic approach to cancer treatment	57
The management of cancer treatment side effects	62
How Camel Milk aids in the recovery from cancer	66
How can friends and family help?	73
Staying cancer free	79
We can win the war on cancer if we:	83
Pay attention to the main causes of cancer	83
Change the approach of western medicine	86
Change how oncology is practised.	89
Appendix A: Blood tests for cancer patients	96
References	103

Forward

The purpose of this book is to give you information so that you can come to your own conclusions. I am telling you about my journey with cancer in the hopes that you can use this information and also experience a remarkable recovery and another chance in life to raise your kids and be awesome.

Your first question when reading this book might be: "What qualifies me to write this book?" I am so glad that you asked. You are precisely the type of reader that this book is written for. The person that questions, that wants to know why. This will be your biggest friend on your road to recovery.

I have been through cancer twice. The first time was in 2013 with breast cancer, where I had a double mastectomy, chemotherapy, and radiation. This was my first personal experience with the dreaded disease. Emotionally there is nothing that can prepare you for this. One day everything is fine. You don't even feel sick at all, and the next moment death is knocking on the door, looking you in the eye and asking you if you are UP for the challenge.

The challenge is not only set to you personally but also to your family and friends. After surviving the first round, I thought: "This is it, I made it". Little did I know that a large portion of first-time cancer survivors will have to deal with this monster again. Statistics made available on the internet suggests that one in six people will have to deal with cancer again. In 2018, it was time for my second encounter when I was diagnosed with stage 4 breast cancer.

Through both these experiences, I was shocked at the attitudes of two of my oncologists; how they would prescribe treatments within a couple of minutes without explaining the treatment plan properly. I also encountered life-threatening mistakes in the administration and management of my treatment. There are some wonderful oncologists out there. *Please* make sure that you are treated by one of them. This will be a big contributing factor in your recovery.

We are dealing with one of the most feared diseases on the planet, and the success rate of conventional cancer treatment does very little to instil confidence in any person. Two things saved my life. Firstly, I listened to my body. Despite what any doctor says, your body will tell you what it can and cannot handle. This led me to leave my first oncologist and to find one that really cares and understands the impact of the treatments on my body. I needed someone that had enough experience with cancer to know that every patient is different and that the patient should rather be a partner in the recovery process and not merely a patient.

Secondly, I read everything about all the medications that they prescribed and challenged them on the fact that the side effects were not adequately explained. There was no way that I could make an informed decision and consent to treatment if I did not have all the information.

This is the key: When you accept the treatment, you consent to it. How can you do this if you don't have all the facts? It is simply impossible. The answer I got every time is that most people will die from cancer and that they do not wish to know about all the side effects. Also, in their opinion, the side effects are not that bad since death is worse. This simply is not true.

What life do you have if you are disabled after the treatment? How do you provide for your family if the cancer treatment has taken away important capabilities? Here I speak from experience. After the wrong administration of my chemotherapy in 2014 (this happens more often than we know) I had severe chemotherapy brain and spent many months after the treatment gaining back my mental capacity.

I have concluded that the average person does not know the first thing about cancer. It scares *us* so much that we refuse to talk or read about it; as if you can contract cancer from reading about it. Western medicine that we have learned to trust so dearly over the last hundred years has failed to come up with a cure and cancer is still listed as an incurable disease. Every sixth death in the world is attributable to some form of cancer. People are too scared to try a different approach because, although the success rate is less than desirable, at least you know what to expect. Better the devil you know.

It is precisely this attitude that has brought the invention of a cancer cure to almost a grinding halt. New chemotherapies are developed, but what we need is an entirely new approach. We need to go back to what cancer is and look at it from a completely different angle. Dare to question, dare to investigate, dare to beat cancer. This is my *mission*.

The only way that cancer can be beaten is through a holistic approach to recovery, where all the aspects of the patients' health are taken into consideration. Most oncologists just treat cancer; this is the biggest problem. There is a huge emotional side to beating cancer and a host of other physical factors to consider.

I hope that this book will become your guide on your road to recovery. I will highlight pitfalls and my experiences throughout the book as well as give advice from the perspective of someone with practical experience of cancer. I want to empower you with information so that you can make your own decisions. It is *your* body, and the responsibility rests with you to look after it.

The other factor that significantly contributes to less effective oncology treatments is that most oncologists have never had cancer. It is like having a mechanic that can't drive. They understand the theory but have no concept of the practical implications of what they do. The medical community has not really found the root cause of cancer; otherwise, they would be able to cure it, and the number of people dying from cancer would be substantially less. They look at commonalities between patients, what do certain groups of patients have in common? But the root cause has been left untouched.

Let's shake the holy establishment that is called the medical profession, where we have been forbidden to enter. Let's question and become part of the complete cure for cancer. Clearly, the medical establishment is unable to find it on their own, so they need our help and our practical guidance for this triumph. There is a single factor that causes cancer; we just need to get to it. This will not be a new discovery and will be found in the existing work of medical professionals and researchers. The answers are already there, we just need to connect the dots and discover the truth about cancer.

If you want to recover from cancer, you need to manage your own therapy, listen to your body and listen to your intuition. If your body tells you it can't take any more chemotherapy, then *listen* to it. To do this, you will need to be brave. You are going to face the ridicule of oncologists, your general practitioner, and scared family and friends. Here lies the first hurdle that we need to cross. Cancer does not equal death. It is feared only because we do not understand what cancer really is. This scares your oncologist, your general practitioner, your family and friends and yourself. Decide this instant that you will recover. You will beat this and become part of the pioneers that will eventually be responsible for a cure for cancer.

You need to know that you cannot trust anyone else with your health than yourself. My experiences with oncologists, who have studied for many years and that have been practising and are *still* practising, was shocking. My first oncologist in 2018 only saw a woman with stage 4 breast cancer, and in her mind, there is no possible cure. So, she gave the standard protocol treatment. She told me that I have two to three years and that I will have to be on chemotherapy for that time.

I'm glad that she told me this because that motivated me to find another way and to do my own research. I was not going to accept the fact that someone wants to put an expiry date on my life. I want you to know what is happening in the medical world, so that you might recognize a problem on your own recovery journey and that you will have time to correct it.

Cancer places an immense strain on relationships. Sometimes you will not feel well and snap. Other times you will feel defeated, and maybe your friends feel locked out. By involving them in your recovery takes a lot of the strain out of the relationships and builds camaraderie. See them as part of your recovery team.

Why this book matters

There are far too many people who needlessly lose their lives to cancer because they don't have proper information about the disease or are prescribed inadequate treatment plans by their doctors. People need to know that cancer is far from a death sentence and that with the right treatment and management of therapy, even some of the most insurmountable odds can be beaten. Obviously, there will be people that get diagnosed far too late for anything to be done, but for the most part, 9.6 million (World Health Organization, 2018) people that lose their lives each year, death could have, and perhaps even should have, been avoided.

One of my biggest aims of this book was to debunk the myth that cancer is unbeatable, and in doing so, remove some of the fear that we so instinctively give rise to whenever the topic comes up. No one wants to think or talk about cancer—of course, they don't. Even when I was diagnosed, I didn't want to talk about cancer. All I wanted to do was disappear and pretend that it didn't exist. The problem with pretending that something doesn't exist though is that when the day comes that you realise it actually does, you're completely unprepared for it—like a deer in the headlights.

When that happens, our first instinct is to look for someone to tell us what to do, blindly placing our trust in anyone wearing a lab coat or holding a doctorate. In any profession, some people excel at what they do, and some don't – make sure that the oncologist you choose excels in their profession. No matter how knowledgeable or trained in their field of expertise doctors maybe, they're not the ones who have been diagnosed with the disease, nor are they the ones who will die if they make a mistake—you are.

To put it quite simply, when it comes to fighting for your life, no one will fight harder than you, and the best way to fight is with knowledge. Although there has been some progress with regards to, for example, immunotherapy research over the years, scientific and medical institutions are still far too resistant in investigating and implementing alternative and complementary treatment methods for cancer.

This needs to change, and while it may be naïve of me to expect this book to be the catalyst to that change, I knew from the moment that I was diagnosed with stage 4 Breast Cancer and placed on palliative care that I needed to at least try. Of course, while I hope that this book will revolutionise the medical world, I at the very least want to know that this book has made a difference in the lives of cancer patients and their families. After all, that difference could be the difference between life and death.

Cancer can be beaten. What cancer will also do, though, is force you to look within yourself and find a level of strength that you never even knew you had.

You can never give up— *I never gave up.*

My own journey with cancer

I first became aware of cancer at a very early age—too early to appreciate the fear which the word commanded. It was my aunt who had just been diagnosed with the disease, and I remember my parents asking me to pray for her. This was my first indication that cancer was something to be taken seriously—something to be feared. It would be some time in the future though before I truly understood the pain of it. This time around, it was my cousin's turn to step into battle. She was 34 when she died, and the day it happened, there was an undeniable sense of relief in the air that her fight was finally over. It was strange to think of death that way. Haunting even. I can only imagine what it must have felt like for her husband and her son, who had to somehow reconcile that relief with the irreplaceable void that would be left in her wake.

For me, her death was a confirmation of that same fear that had been suggested upon me as a small child. It would continue to grow years later when a classmate of my daughter was diagnosed. She was only a small child herself at the time—only eleven when she died. I remember trying to explain what had happened to my daughter of the same age, but how could I when I still didn't even understand it myself?

By then, there was so much publicity surrounding cancer and how deadly it was, that when it was eventually my turn to be diagnosed, all I could think about was the inevitability of my own death. The truth is, I didn't actually know anything else about cancer. All I knew was that it killed and that it did so indiscriminately.

My first cancer diagnosis.

I was diagnosed with breast cancer on the 9th of December 2013. The day before was a Sunday, and I had woken up that morning to what I had believed to be a perfect life. I had a dream job, loving husband, two wonderful children, and all the means to support them with. The only thing that I could still rightly ask for, in this perfect life of mine, was more time for me to enjoy it.

I was very passionate about my job, but the hours were demanding, which meant that regularly, I was either out of town or out of the country and away from my husband and children. My family means everything to me, and so it broke my heart every time I missed one of my daughter's gymnastics competitions or one of my son's tennis tournaments. The worst part was thinking that it broke their hearts too, which is why Riaan (my husband) and I had made plans that December to enjoy a much needed and deserved holiday with our beautiful children, Alexandra and JJ.

Little did any of us know how quickly and how dramatically those plans were about to change. On Sunday morning, 8 December, I got up out of bed and made breakfast for my family. The children had playdates with their friends that day, and I was going to catch up on some work. It seemed, by all means, a pretty run of the mill, non-exceptional Sunday. Of course, it's on those seemingly non-exceptional days where one's life always seems to take a turn for the worst.

For me, that turn started when my husband detected a lump in my breast—a glitch in my perfect life. Given my family's history with cancer, the discovery was quite disconcerting for me, but I didn't let it show. In fact, I dismissed it as if the lump weren't even there, hoping that it was only as real as I made it out to be. My husband was far less cavalier, though, which only added to the anxiety that was secretly stirring inside of me.

The next day, I met with my general practitioner and told him about the lump. After examining me, he said that he didn't think it was cancerous, but he didn't want to take any chances. I was sent for a mammogram and a biopsy, the results of which would only be revealed to me later that day. I remember feeling quite relieved as I stepped out of the consulting room—optimistic even. I thought to myself that the doctor wouldn't get my hopes up about the lump not being cancerous unless he was sure that it wasn't.

I shared the good news with my husband as soon as I got the chance. He sounded relieved too. A few hours later, at around five, I received a phone call from the doctor's office, telling me that my results were in and that I needed to see my doctor right away. I was at work at the time, but immediately stopped what I was doing and rushed back over to his consulting room as quickly as I could.

I think I knew before he told me. I could see the anguish on his face. It was like he was trying to work up the courage to look his dog in the eye before putting a bullet in its head. There was no dog around though. There was just me, and despite being able to see the bullet coming from a mile away, I could do nothing to avoid it. All I could do was wait for it to hit. "Mrs Brazer, I am so sorry…but you have cancer, and it's rather serious," he told me.

I felt numb as I heard the words, and then paralysed, and then altogether detached as if I was watching this all unfold from outside my body. The doctor and I both had tears in our eyes. "Will I make it?" I eventually found the courage to ask.

He told me that my oncologist would have to do further testing before we could confirm that I was about to die. He didn't quite say it like that, but that's how I heard it. Any response other than him telling me I would survive was going to feel like a death sentence. And so, in my unfeeling, detached state, with tears still running down my eyes, I gave a nod to show that I understood, lifted myself up out of my seat, and then calmly left the room.

I was having the worst moment of my life, and now I had to go home and somehow find the strength to share that moment with the three people who I loved most in the world. It was unthinkable. I just sat there in my car in the parking lot, unable to move, let alone drive. Inevitably, the numbness gave way to the pain, and I burst into tears, sobbing uncontrollably as the reality of my situation started to sink in. I knew that the pain was far too great for me to deal with on my own, and so I started the car and drove home to my family.

The drive home was both the longest and shortest of my life. The garage door opened as I arrived, and my husband and children were waiting for me on the other side, waving excitedly. I felt my heart shatter as soon as I saw them. Later that evening, the four of us were all sitting around the dining room table when my husband began to explain to the children why I had been crying. I was unable to utter a single word, still reeling from the shock of the news. As soon as my daughter heard him say *cancer*, she became hysterical.

"Mommy is going to die," she said.

My husband tried to console her, but she insisted that cancer would kill me, just as it had killed her classmate the previous year. I believed it too. My ten-year-old son then grabbed onto me and pleaded with me not to die. I was as desperate for that not to happen as they were but felt helpless to stop it. We did our best to come to terms with my diagnosis as a family, but for the most part of that evening, there were just tears.

Towards the end of it, as my husband was on the phone with family, I went outside and sat down on the porch. My mind was still racing, and I was in no state to speak to anyone. As I was staring out over my garden with tears still in my eyes, I started to wonder what would happen to my husband and kids if I died.

They weren't ready to lose me, and I wasn't ready to be lost. There was still so much I wanted to do with my life, and now suddenly so little time to do it in. What mattered most? How could I make my final days worthwhile? These were the sort of impossible questions that formed and fell apart in my head throughout that night. Eventually, I lost my strength to think entirely and went off to bed. I was so drained from all the crying and worrying, that I fell asleep almost as soon as my head hit the pillow. And that was the end of day one.

Tuesday morning came—it was the day of our office Christmas Party. I was in no mood for people, but I pieced myself together anyway in the hope of a distraction. When I arrived in the parking lot, my secretary was there waiting for me with tears in her eyes. After giving me a much-needed hug, I asked her not to tell anyone else as I did not want to ruin the party. I had an appointment with my surgeon that same day, and so, about forty-five minutes into the party, I excused myself and drove over to his consulting room.

My surgeon informed me that the tumour needed to be removed and then went about explaining the procedure to me and how they would attempt to save my breast. It was at that point (with the little knowledge of cancer I had) that I insisted that he perform a mastectomy and remove the breast entirely. My decision was based on the understanding that if I had no breast, then cancer couldn't come back. It then occurred to me that I might one day have the same problem with the other breast, so I doubled down on my decision and asked that he remove them both. The idea was that if I somehow survived this war with cancer, then I sure as hell wasn't going to take any chance of having to go through it again. My surgery was scheduled for 17 December 2013.

Upon my return to the Christmas party, it was clear to everyone in attendance that I was out of sorts. I may as well have been wearing a big neon sign with 'cancer' written across my chest. I didn't say anything until the formalities commenced and it was my turn, as the director of my division, to address and thank my staff for all their tireless work and contributions over the last year.

My speech started with "I am so proud of my team…" I broke down in tears before I could complete the thought. The only words I could muster after that were, "I have been diagnosed with cancer." I then sat down and tried to regather myself while my line manager explained my situation to the rest of the room. For the rest of the day, my friends and colleagues, one by one, all offered me their deep-felt sympathies and support.

It was now six days to go until the first operation of my life. I had never been under anaesthesia before and had a hellish fear that I wasn't going to wake up afterwards. As if that wasn't enough to deal with, I now also had to contend with the never-ending flood of phone calls from friends and family, letting me know that they were thinking of me and that I needed to be strong. I appreciated the support, but every time someone told me that they were thinking about me, it meant that I was thinking about me too, and by extension, my cancer.

The more real it became, the more I started to wonder if these were the last six days of my life. The thought that kept playing on repeat in my mind was, "What can I teach my kids in these next six days that will prepare them for the rest of their lives?" The simple answer was *nothing*.

It wasn't that I didn't have any wisdom to share with them, but rather that it was impossible for me to articulate that wisdom in a way that they might understand. I even considered writing them birthday cards for all the years of their lives that I would miss, but the problem was the same – you can't prepare for life. You can only react to it, and the ability to do so is not something that can be taught, but something that must be learned through experience. I could never teach them wisdom like that in a million years, let alone six days. I could only pray that they would find that wisdom somewhere along the way, as I did.

17 December—The day of my operation. I entered the hospital at 07:30 a.m. with my husband and my kids. After checking in, we were escorted to my ward, and I was given a theatre gown to change into. I remember sitting there in the hospital bed with my bra in my hand and thinking to myself that I was never going to have to wear one of these again. At peace with the thought, I tossed the bra into the dustbin and then readied myself as best I could for what was to come.

The anaesthesiologist met with my family and me soon after. He was kind to my kids and explained to us that I would feel nothing once he administered the anaesthesia. It then came time for me to be wheeled into theatre. My husband and kids followed me to the doors where I kissed them goodbye. I remember fearing that that was going to be the last time I would ever see them again. I also remember what the inside of the theatre looked like and the coldness I felt when I transferred myself from the bed to the operating table. I was asked to count backward from ten while the anaesthesia was being administered. I faded to black before I even got started and then for the next 3 hours—nothing.

When I woke up, I was back in the ward. There was a nurse at my bedside. She was adjusting my drip as my family watched on from the foot of the bed. Everything between then and the day I got to go home is a painkiller-induced haze. I remember my best friend since grade 1, Retha, coming to visit me in the days that followed. She was always the first person I would phone when I needed help and given that she had studied nursing when she was younger meant that she could assist in the cleaning out of my drainage pumps. Her help and expertise during this difficult time were much appreciated, as was the love and support from the rest of my friends and family.

24 December 2013. My children quietly entered my room to wish me Happy Birthday. I don't remember what they got me, but I do remember that we were all crying as they sang to me. I turned 43 that day and slept through most of it thanks to a robust prescription of pain medication. Before I knew it, it was already Christmas, and then New Year.

We decided to have a party that night. It would be the first of a new tradition in our family —a tradition where we celebrate every special occasion as if it were our last. A week or so later, I saw my surgeon again. He told me that he was happy with how the wound was healing, and I could begin with chemotherapy in February. As I was going to lose my hair, I decided that I was going to beat it to the punch and get my head shaved. My husband and my son did the same, as a show of solidarity. If we were going to get through this, we were going to do it together, as a family.

In early February 2014, I underwent chemotherapy for the first time. My oncologist told me that day that if I wanted to survive, I needed to do exactly as he said. I was scared beyond words. I weighed 66 kilograms at the time and needed to be closely monitored because there was a very real possibility that my body wouldn't be able to handle the full dosage.

I sat there in the chemotherapy room for two hours and five IV bags in total.

The chemotherapy itself was a bright red liquid. I felt awful by the time I got home. I didn't feel like eating anything and spent about two days in bed before my husband decided to rush me to my GP. By then, I was bending over the toilet four to five times a day and losing weight rapidly. My GP immediately put me on an IV drip, and I soon felt better.

My condition continued to improve throughout the next three weeks until it was time for round two of chemotherapy. It was even worse this time. I could hardly keep anything in when I got home, and my mouth tasted like metal. The next morning, I woke up with excruciating stomach cramps and desperately needed the bathroom. By lunchtime that day, I needed to be rushed to my GP again. He gave me another IV drip and some tablets for the stomach cramps.

Two hellish days later and I was back again. I remember waking up and finding my son lying on the floor next to my bed with a pillow and a blanket. He looked up at me and said, "Please, mommy, you can't die now, I still need to learn from you. There are so many things I don't know."

After that, I informed my husband I wanted to stop the treatment. I was certain that the chemotherapy was going to kill me anyway, and I didn't want my children to remember me like that. My husband burst into tears when I told him this. "You cannot give up, you have to fight this," he pleaded with me.

I told him that the only way I would reconsider was if he could find me a better oncologist. And so, that's what he did. The next day, when I returned to my oncologist's practice for my medical file, the receptionist informed me that it was their property and that I would be wasting both my time and money by going elsewhere. Quite irritated by the comment, I asked to speak to my oncologist personally but was told that he was busy and could not see me. That made me furious, so I decided to place a phone call to the Health Professions Council of South Africa and asked them for their assistance.

A few moments later and the receptionist ushered me into the oncologists' office. He wanted to know why I wanted to go to another oncologist and claimed that he was not aware that I had any problems with my treatments, despite me insisting weeks prior that my nausea medication was not working. I reminded him of this and then insisted that he give me my medical file. At that point, people in the reception area were starting to stare, but I wasn't going to move until I had my file.

My first appointment with my new oncologist coincided with my third chemotherapy session. After studying my file very closely, he looked up at me and asked, "What antidepressants are you currently using?" The question came as a surprise to me as I had not been using antidepressants at the time. I told him this, and he looked equally surprised. As it turned out, the nausea medication that I had been prescribed by my previous oncologist depression as a side effect.

His next question was: "What supplements are you currently using?" Again, I told him that I was not using any supplements because my previous oncologist forbade it due to the fact that it could make the chemotherapy less effective. He told me that at the very least, I should have been taking Vitamin C to assist my immune system as he could see from the GP's records that I had been sick a couple of times already.

He then asked me to explain to him why I wanted to stop with the therapy and what specific side effects caused me to make this decision. The list was long. It included memory loss, rapidly deteriorating eyesight, constant nausea, fatigue, breathlessness, and an inability to hold any food down. Most concerning was that I had already lost 20 kilograms in only eight weeks. After hearing all this, my oncologist asked me if I would be willing to continue with the treatment if he were able to diminish the aforementioned symptoms. I said that I would and then, a few moments later, was escorted to the chemotherapy room for my third session.

What immediately caught my attention when the nurse re-entered the chemotherapy room, was that she was carrying a rather a big bag of orange liquid. When I asked her what was inside the bag, a confused expression came over her. She then asked me if I had ever undergone chemotherapy before. I told her that I had, but that in my first two sessions, I was treated with a much smaller bag containing a bright red liquid. The colour drained from her face as she heard this. A few moments later, she returned to the room with my oncologist, and he then asked me to describe to him exactly what my chemotherapy bags looked like.

To his shock, the bright red colour that I had described to him was undiluted chemotherapy, which, according to him, was responsible for 90% of the side-effects that I had described just moments prior. On my way home that day, I was not nearly as tired as I usually was and for the first time in a while, I began to feel hope again that I could come out on the other side of this war alive.

I kept thinking about the chemotherapy that I received at my previous oncologist and couldn't help but wonder about all the other patients who have had to endure the same hell as I did and whose lives may presently still be in danger due to this practice. My conscience wouldn't allow me to let the issue lie, so I decided to phone the Health Professions Council of South Africa again to enquire further into the matter.

After explaining to the lady on the other end of the phone what had happened, she quite insensitively responded by telling me that there was nothing that they could do and that I should just be grateful to be alive. This was shocking to hear from an institution whose primary purpose is to ensure that such issues are brought to light and dealt with. I told her that if she did not want to attend to my complaint, I would take it to the media and maybe that would inspire them to take the matter more seriously.

Within two days, I received a call back from them to tell me that they had investigated the issue and had put measures in place to ensure that the chemotherapy would be given in accordance with the best treatment practices. After being made to feel so small and weak by cancer, it was empowering for me to know that I still had a voice and that I was able to use it to make some sort of difference in the world, even if it was in a small way.

In the days leading up to my final chemotherapy session, I felt a considerable improvement in my condition, and thanks to the Vitamin C supplement that I had been prescribed, I had not been sick once since switching oncologists. Things were undoubtedly starting to look up.

During that final session, we discussed how to go about my radiation treatment. It was not practical for me to do it there as my new oncologist was situated 300 kilometres out from where we lived, and I would need to make myself available for treatment five days a week for the next six weeks. Knowing this, I insisted that he write a letter specifying in detail how my treatment needed to be handled so that a situation like the one with my previous oncologist could be avoided. He was uncomfortable prescribing for another doctor, but he understood my concerns and wrote the letter anyway.

Upon receiving the said letter, my new doctors were not exactly thrilled about being prescribed to, but I made it quite clear to them that if they did not apply the treatment exactly as instructed in the letter, I would report them. Fortunately, there was no need for that, and my treatment could proceed without any more drama. The radiation sessions were overall very successful, and a month later, my cancer was in remission. I had won the war.

My second cancer diagnosis

The four years following my cancer diagnosis were extremely difficult, both professionally and personally. Despite having beaten cancer, my life was now far from perfect, and the stress that I was carrying was, in my opinion, what ultimately led to my second diagnosis.

The signs started somewhere in April of 2017. I injured my hip while attempting a ballet exercise. The incident left me in extreme discomfort, which I tried to remedy with painkillers and a couple of days' rest. When that didn't work, I made an appointment with a chiropractor who, after evaluating my hip, sent me for x-rays. The scans revealed that I had incurred a not-so-serious injury known as an *impingement,* which was quickly sorted out with two weeks of therapy.

In June 2018 the pain returned. This was right before we were about to go on holiday, so I decided that instead of attending to the issue right away, as I should have, I was rather going to stock up on some pain medication and then see a doctor again when we got back. I worked in retail distribution at the time, which meant that openings for a holiday were few and far between. With good planning and a bit of luck, however, we were able to carve out six days at the end of June to spend some quality time, and I wasn't about to forgo that precious time with *my* family for a little niggle in my hip. So, I powered through the pain and went on holiday with my now ex-husband and children, hoping that I would be back to my old self again after a day or two at the sea.

It had been a long time since we had been to our holiday house. When we arrived, the first thing the kids did was run down to the beach. I couldn't really walk all that well at that point, so I decided to stay behind on the porch for the first day. It didn't get easier the next day, or the day after that, so I decided to see a doctor while I was down there (East London).

I hobbled into the consultation room on the morning of July 2nd using my daughter's old crutches that I had brought along on the trip in case I needed them. The doctor was an elderly gentleman— very old school in his approach. He said that he wanted to examine me properly before he recommended a method of treatment. Noticing that my back was skew (due to a horse-riding accident in high school), he decided it was best for me to get x-rays taken.

It would still be another hour before I could see him again about the results, so my family and I decided to get something to eat while we waited, completely oblivious to how our lives were about to change yet again. When the hour had passed, we returned to the doctor's office. I had so much difficulty walking that my ex-husband needed to push me into the consultation room in a wheelchair.

Once we both sat down, the doctor looked to me and asked, "Why didn't you tell me that you had breast cancer before?" The question caught me off guard. "How do you know that I had cancer before? And what does that have to do with my hip pain?" I asked.

He then slowly turned his computer monitor around so that we could see the x-rays for ourselves. To my horror, my hip and back looked like Swiss cheese. And that's when he said it, "You have stage 4 breast cancer, Nina. I am so sorry."

It took me a moment to process what I had just heard. It felt like a blade had just been plunged into the pit of my stomach. "How bad is it?" I asked. "Well, it's bad enough that you have to leave for your hometown immediately and get to an oncologist as soon as possible," he answered before proceeding to drive the blade in even deeper. "Stage 4 breast cancer is treatable, but not curable. I am very sorry."

And just like that, the world stopped moving again. I was paralysed in the chair, asking myself and anyone brave enough to answer, "Why is this happening again? Why is this happening to me again?" No one answered.

The next thing the doctor told me was that with the right therapy, I could live a couple of years more. Can you imagine that? A couple of years. With the right therapy…I could live a couple of years. I just sat there, stone-faced as tears rolled down my cheeks. Our children were waiting in the reception area as this was all happening and when we came out of the consultation room, my son, who was now fifteen, asked me, "Mommy, what did the doctor say?"

I tried to keep the tears back as I told him that my hip was broken. "Thank God it's not cancer," he replied. That was when I lost all control and began to sob like a child. His dad explained to him that my hip was broken because the cancer was back, and it was eating away at my bones. My daughter's expression matched the horror of the description. "Are you going to die, Mommy?" she asked me.

"Yes," I told her, "but not now—the doctors can give me treatment, so I have another year or two. "It was harder for me to say the words than it was for me to hear them. The question quickly stopped being, "Why is this happening to me again?" and became, "Why is this happening to them again?" And still, no one answered.

The drive home was brutal, filled with long and uncomfortable silences between every failed attempt at normality. As mentioned before, it hadn't been an easy four years as it was. This holiday came at a time when it was desperately needed. My cancer diagnosis, though, not so much.

"We have to tell your family," said my ex-husband. "I can't…I don't want to talk to anyone right now. Can you do it, please?"

When we got back to the holiday house, we all sat down on the porch and started to cry together. The kids went down to the beach later that afternoon to say goodbye to the sea, and when my son came back, he was holding a bucket. He gave it to me and said, "Mommy, here is the sea. There is sand, a fishy, shells…" He started to cry again as he explained that he had brought me the sea in a bucket because I was never going to be able to see it again.

If I wasn't broken before, I was now. I don't remember much about the journey home except for my ex-husband asking me if I wanted him to stay at the house to assist me. It was a kind and generous offer, which I gratefully accepted.

My appointment with my new oncologist was set for Thursday. After sending me for a quick scan and some blood tests, she confirmed that all I could hope for was two to three years. The number was assuming all went well, however, and in my case, all going *well* required me to be on chemotherapy for those two or three years which meant the remainder of my life. She also said that they would try and restore my mobility with Zoledronic acid (a drug used to treat bone disease) and that I would need to start radiation immediately to prevent further fractures.

She had me placed on very strong painkillers (Tramacet) and sent me home to rest before my first session. I made sure to do my research on Zoledronic acid and find out exactly how it should be administered. I didn't want a repeat of what happened in 2014, where medications were administered incorrectly.

I also Googled everything I could about stage 4 breast cancer, hoping to find some slither of hope that I could hang onto. Every result came back the same though—*Treatable, but not curable*. I couldn't accept this. I wasn't just going to rot in palliative care for the next two years, waiting to die. If I was going down, then I was going down swinging. I needed to find just one person that has fully recovered from stage 4 cancer…I desperately needed this hope.

Exhausted after my first radiation session, I went straight home and slept. I woke up nauseated and feeling extremely unwell. The following morning, I woke up feeling even worse, so my oncologist put me on an IV drip before my next radiation session to counter nausea. That didn't help relieve my symptoms, and later that afternoon, I was beset with stomach cramps and spasms so intense that I felt my ribcage contracting.

After being rushed to the emergency room, the doctor that attended to me said that the pain was emanating from a stomach ulcer which I had developed as a result of all the painkillers I'd taken. The medication he gave me to treat the ulcer didn't help with my symptoms either, which persisted well past my third radiation session the following day.

When I got home, I lay down in the sunroom. My family had converted it into a temporary bedroom for me to rest in during the day. This was much appreciated—I didn't want to be shrouded in darkness all the time and found it comforting to be able to stare out at my garden.

By the next day, my stomach cramps still hadn't gone away, so I was prescribed another IV drip. This was also the day I was due to start with my Zolodronic Acid treatment. The problem, however, was that I only had one viable arm for drawing blood and inserting IV's. The nurse thought it would be a good idea to administer my nausea medication and Zoledronic acid using the same IV drip. Based on the research I had done on Zoledronic acid, I knew that this was something which simply should not be done.

I immediately brought it to the attention of the attending doctor, who to my shock, saw nothing wrong with the way my treatment was being administered. I proceeded to show him the literature which I had researched, to which he responded by saying, "Oh well then, just take the nausea medication, and we'll give you the Zoledronic acid once you're done with radiation."

I was quite thrown by his nonchalant attitude towards my health. It was as if he either had no awareness of the horrible mistake that was almost made, or he just didn't care. Such incompetence and negligence are not acceptable in any profession, let alone one where you're responsible for other people's lives.

As I sat there with the IV dripping away, I received an unexpected phone call from one of my suppliers. I answered, expecting to receive condolences but was instead given something far better—hope. He said that I needed to speak to his mother, explaining to me that she was diagnosed with stage 4 cancer too and had been cured for 8 years already. I couldn't believe what I was hearing. It was like music to my ears. I needed to speak to this woman and find out how she was still alive.

I did so, later that afternoon, over the phone. The journey which she described to me was long, painstaking, and very expensive. This left me in a bit of a predicament as my medical insurance would not cover the costs. I had no other option but to sell my business. I was reluctant to do this. I had only started it up again the previous year, and my financial situation was just beginning to look up again. But I had no choice. I had to do whatever I could to keep myself alive. So, in order to finance my recovery, I closed the business and liquidated my assets. I thought that if I could get this done in a year, then I might just be okay. It was a big ask, but I had overcome great challenges before and was determined to overcome even more.

That same afternoon, I decided to try and ride out my stomach pain and ate very small portions of food to try and negate nausea. The next day, I was put on yet another IV drip, and just like the ones before, it did nothing to relieve my symptoms. I was back in the emergency room later that night. I was told that my ulcer medication was not working (a fact I was already painfully aware of) and was then given new medication and sent home again. At the time, I was drinking eight Tramacet tablets a day—two before even lifting my head from the pillow in the mornings.

After my fifth radiation session, I couldn't take it anymore and decided to go back to my old oncologist, who was now located even further out from my home—700 kilometres in total. Just like the last time, attaining my medical file from the oncologist was a nightmare. Also, just like the last time, the issue was resolved with another call to the Health Professions Council of South Africa.

After all that, I was finally back with my old oncologist. We drove up to see him the following morning. I was quite excited about the trip and even hopeful that he had better news for me than what the other doctors and Google had been giving me. I walked into his office on crutches, medical files in hand. He smiled at me as I entered and then asked, "How can I help you today?" I smiled back and said, "If you could cure my stomach pain, that would be a good start."

I was sent for x-rays, and that's where we realised what the problem was. I was so blocked up from all the pain tablets I had been taking that nothing could fit any more. I couldn't believe that it had taken this long to figure out what was wrong with me. Surely two different GP's and an oncologist should have been able to pick this up sooner. In any case, I was thrilled that the cause of my stomach pain had been detected and was eager to move on with my treatment.

Travelling 700 km back and forth every three weeks was still not a viable option though, so I was recommended yet another oncologist in my hometown. My only request was that my old oncologist finds me, someone, who was as good at their job as he was, and who also cared about their patients as much as he did.

All in all, it was a good trip. The only negative was that when I asked him about my odds of surviving cancer, he repeated what almost everyone else had already said—that I would likely die.

Five radiation sessions later, and I was finally done. After my final session, I told my oncologist that I would not be continuing my treatment with her. The reason I gave her was that it felt like I was just another patient to her and that she didn't really care about my well-being at all. She responded by telling me that she had too many patients to give us all individualised attention. I didn't stick around for too long after I heard that. I knew that if I was going to have any hope of surviving cancer this time around, I couldn't be relying on the so-called expertise of doctors who didn't even see me as a real person.

No, this was my life—my fight. If I was going to overcome the odds again, I had to take matters into my own hands. I decided to start by doing more cancer research, focusing specifically on what cancer is, how it grows, and how it dies. The problem was that I have no medical or science background, but somehow, I had to grasp the science behind it. Realising that I needed to become better acquainted with my enemy, I adjusted my search to the most fundamental question I could think of—

What is cancer?

According to Cancer.net, "Cells grow and divide to make new cells as the body needs them. Usually, cells die when they get too old or damaged. Then, new cells take their place. Cancer begins when genetic changes interfere with this orderly process." This was my first clue— *cancer forms at cellular level.*

When I met with my new oncologist, the first thing she asked me when I gave her my medical file was, "Where is the rest of it?" I told her that that was all that there was, and she looked at me with a puzzled expression. She said that it was not possible to prescribe a proper treatment plan with the little information that was in the file and that she needed to know more about me to be able to establish a proper baseline with which she could track my progress.

When she said this, I couldn't help but think about my previous oncologist who took one look at me and decided, without any consideration for who I was as a person, that my death was inevitable. She treated me as if I were an exercise in a textbook, rather than a mother of two children who was fighting for her life.

Altogether, the appointment took about 45 minutes, whereas my intake session with my first oncologist barely took ten. When we were done, I went home and waited for her to call me and advise me on possible treatments. I was strolling around the garden on my crutches when I received the call. She told me that my cancer count (CA 15-3) had doubled in the last three weeks and that I needed to undergo chemotherapy again.

Not wanting the same disastrous results as the first time, I decided to research if there was something that I could take, which could help my body cope with the chemotherapy. Vitamin C was an obvious choice, but I also stumbled upon a powerful antioxidant called GHS, which is specially formulated for quick absorbency.

That's when I read about camel milk and learned how it was not only an immune booster but that it was especially effective in helping cancer patients to cope with the side-effects of chemotherapy. The chemotherapy that my oncologist decided on for me was Xeloda. The side effects are as follows:

- Severe nausea and vomiting.
- Stomach pain.
- Loss of appetite.
- Constipation.
- Tiredness and fatigue.
- Pain in the back, joints, and muscles.
- Severe headaches.
- Dizziness.
- Difficulty sleeping.
- Darkened spots on the skin.
- Dryness, itchiness, and rashes.
- Numbness and/or tingling in hands and feet.
- Temporary nail changes, including fungal infections.

I insisted that I wouldn't be taking a full dose of chemotherapy due to the disaster that was my previous experience, and I would rather monitor my progress through my cancer counts every three weeks.

I also shared with her what I had learned about camel milk, specifically about how it's been shown to assist in the healing of bones. She seemed surprised. I told her that I would only be willing to use the Zoledronic acid until I could walk again. She looked at me with an empathetic smile and said, "That might be a while still."

When I got home later that day, I immediately opened my laptop and started searching for camel milk in South Africa. To my surprise and delight, there was actually a camel dairy in the country. I spoke with the man who owned the farm. His name was Hans—and yes, he milked camels. I told him that I had stage 4 breast cancer and that I wanted to use the camel milk to help with my recovery. He was sceptical that it would work but took my order anyway.

A week later, and my first box of milk arrived. I had no idea what the recommended dosage was, so I started out with 250 millilitres a day. I had already started with chemotherapy by that time and been spending most days in bed, only really getting up to go to the bathroom. Within a week of taking the milk though, I found that the fatigue and lethargy were gone. It wasn't long after that I started venturing out into the garden again. I found that being around my plants and vegetables significantly improved my mood, so I started going out daily.

After two weeks of chemotherapy, it was now time to test my cancer count. My first count was 388. It doubled three weeks later to 734, and now, it was at 1168. Although the rate at which it was growing had slowed down somewhat, my oncologist was still very worried. Quite worried myself, I decided to up my dosage of camel milk to 500ml a day.

The increased intake made a considerable difference as I was now far more energetic than before and was even able to help around the house a bit. Regrettably, though, I was soon brought back down to earth again with another painful reminder of my mortality. It happened as I was helping my daughter clean her room. I was in the process of moving a small cupboard so that I could lay a cloth over the top, and as I was doing this, I felt my chest crack.

The pain was excruciating; I couldn't breathe. After another trip to the hospital, I would find out that I had broken three ribs as well as my pelvis superior. Even worse than the physical pain I was in, was the realisation of how weak my bones really were. I had just started to feel like I was getting my strength back again, and then before I knew it, I was a cripple in a wheelchair. I was shattered inside, quite literally, but I still insisted on getting outside once a day. Even with my children having to push me around in a wheelchair, being in the garden with them gave me something to smile about and reminded me that I was still alive.

After the incident with the cupboard, I decided to up the camel milk dosage to 750ml a day. I needed to walk before my birthday in December. It was only three months away, and my school's thirty-year reunion was also planned for the month before. I had been looking forward to it for some time, and I was determined to be there on my own two feet. In the meantime, I diligently continued my cancer research.

I wanted to know what the difference was between a normal cell and a cancer cell. The terminology was rather technical, and as I did not have a background in science, it was quite difficult for me to make sense of what I was reading. This wasn't a problem, though. I just Googled my way through every word I didn't understand until eventually, I figured out how the energy generation process of cells worked. This would be my second clue—*cancer cells ferment and normal cells respirate.*

Three weeks later and the tide turned. My cancer count was now down to 766. I was winning. I monitored my chemotherapy dosage closely and lowered it as my count was coming down to ease any undue strain on my body. Soon, I was able to start doing things for myself again. This was important and gave me hope that I was going to go all the way and beat this thing.

Back during my first week of chemotherapy, I experienced very dry skin, and it seemed as though all the moisturiser in the world wasn't going to make a difference. It then occurred to me, as I was doing my research on camel milk, that I could use the milk to create some sort of makeshift solution to my problem. I already had lanolin cream lying around, so I decided to combine it with some of the milk and apply it to my body. Although far from elegant, the solution proved highly effective, doing wonders for my skin.

This also helped me to realise that I wanted to venture into skincare as a profession once I recovered from cancer. It was quite shocking to me to realise just how many popular skincare products are made with harmful ingredients, and I thought to myself that I would begin formulating my own natural creams to help people such as myself.

I reacted well to the chemotherapy, and the best part was that I had no side-effects whatsoever. I was feeling good, so much so that I was able to start dressing myself again. I even took trips to the shops with my daughter. I had an automatic car, so driving wasn't too much of a problem. Getting in and out of the car, on the other hand, proved to be slightly more complicated, especially with people giving my daughter and me strange looks in the parking lot when my wheelchair appeared.

But it didn't bother me. I was just happy to be somewhere other than my room or the hospital. At this stage, my cancer count was down to 594, and I could smell victory. The chairperson of my school's reunion committee also phoned me during this time and asked why I hadn't been attending the meetings. Not many people knew about my cancer at this point, and they were all quite shocked when I told them. One of my best friends from high school was especially taken aback by the news. She came to visit me sometime before the reunion and was lost for words when she discovered that I was in a wheelchair. After telling her about my condition, we spent the rest of the day catching up with one another.

Although my cancer count was dropping rapidly, I was still very much invested in my research of the disease and made a fascinating discovery about the link between cancer and oxidative stress. According to Reuter et al. (2010), "Cancer initiation and progression has been linked to oxidative stress by increasing DNA mutations or inducing DNA damage, genome instability, and cell proliferation." I came across many other articles that supported the connection, but interestingly found nothing of the sort on any cancer website that I visited apart from one - the Kresser Institute in Switzerland. I knew that I was on the right track and decided to keep digging deeper.

Towards the end of October, one Saturday morning, I decided that I was going to start walking again. I was determined that this would be the day, so I set my feet down on the floor and cautiously stood up out of bed. Once I saw that I could support my own weight, I took a step forward, and then another, and another. The bathroom was about seven metres away, but I got there in what felt like ten, using the wall as a crutch so that I wouldn't fall.

My son caught sight of me as I passed him in the hallway. "Mom, what are you doing?" he asked in shock. Very proudly, I replied, "I am walking."

I pushed myself to walk a little further every day after that, and by the next Saturday when it was time to go to my reunion, not only was I able to enter on my own two feet, but I even managed to break out a move or two on the dancefloor. It was a great night. The next Monday, I was able to enter the chemotherapy room without any assistance whatsoever. My oncologist, as well as all the nurses that were there, were absolutely gobsmacked that I was walking again. I told her that this was going to be my last day on the Zoledronic acid, and it was.

Even though I had been making remarkable progress, I still couldn't walk more than 200 metres at a time or climb the stairs. It wasn't because I had any pain, but rather that I needed to build up my stamina again after being in a wheelchair for two months. I had always been a very active person, and so, for me to spend so much time sitting around, giving instructions and asking for help was immensely frustrating.

But that was in the past now, and by the time my birthday came around in December, I was back to normal. I could walk, I could run, I could climb, I could garden—I could do *anything*. I even decided to take up ballet again, buying myself a new pink pair of shoes in celebration of my recovery and my victory.

My December count came in at 129, which was slightly more than what it was in November (107). This was when I decided to stop with the chemotherapy. My friends and family pleaded with me not to, but my decision remained unchanged. I just didn't think it was necessary anymore. My research indicated that the camel milk would be all that I need at this stage. Continuing with chemotherapy would do more harm than good.

Trusting my intuition proved to be the correct decision, as by February 2019 my cancer count was down to 83. I also learned a few more interesting facts about cancer during this period, including how the growth of the disease is accelerated by iron and that the lactoferrin in the camel milk that I was drinking was not only removing the iron from my body but also countering the oxidative stress caused by the chemotherapy. This was a big reason why my body responded so well.

By June 2019, my count had been cut in half to 41. This was quite surprising considering that my stress levels were very high at the time. Things had slowed down considerably in terms of my finances, and I was under a lot of pressure to provide for my family. The fact that my levels were still dropping despite all the anxiety I was experiencing is a true testament to the potency of camel milk. It also made it all the more baffling to me how so few people, doctors included, were actually aware of this. That's when I realised that it was my responsibility to start spreading the word. And so, an idea occurred to me—*why not write a book about it*?

What I have learned on my journey and wish I knew before being diagnosed with cancer

After I was placed on palliative care, which was a less than desirable prognosis, I knew that if I wanted to survive cancer, it is going to be up to me to do it. I had to take responsibility and find a way to cure my cancer. My first step was to find out what cancer is.

I had such a desire to live that I did not leave any stone unturned in my search for scientific facts and information about cancer. To fight cancer, I needed to understand how cancer starts, how it grows and, most importantly, how it dies.

The purpose of this chapter is not to explain in detail what cancer is. I want to give you enough information so that you question the therapy that you receive and make your own decisions about your therapy. This will provide you with a definite edge for surviving cancer.

My quest goes beyond this. I will not rest until we have a different approach to cancer therapy worldwide, and people do not die from cancer in droves like they currently do. Where everybody has failed, I must succeed.

What is cancer?

Without having to relay to you my whole study and research journey, I would like to share some highlights with you. I had to start somewhere, and my first question was:

What are the characteristics of cancer cells? Typical hallmarks of the acquired capabilities of tumour cells during tumorigenesis include sustained proliferation, evasion of growth suppressors, resisting cell death, replicative immortality, activating invasion, metastasis, evading the immune system, and reprogramming energy metabolism.

What is the difference between a cancer cell and a normal cell?

It took me more than a month of intense studying before I could answer this one fundamental question. The simple difference between a cancer cell and a normal cell is the way that they produce energy. I studied the whole energy generation cycle of cells to see where the difference lies. Following each part of the process meticulously, I came to my conclusion: Healthy cells use respiration to produce energy and cancer cells use fermentation to produce energy. The first person that made this discovery was Otto Warburg.

Cancer is not a genetic disease

This was my second discovery. According to Prof. Thomas Seyfried, a researcher focusing on cancer, the current dogma that cancer is a genetic disease, this is taught in all the handbooks, so we have indoctrinated several generations of scientists and physicians that every cancer starts with a mutation in a cell nucleus. This belief was already challenged in 1969 and 1975. In 2003 more research was done that confirmed that the evidence does not support the somatic mutation theory (that cancer is a genetic disease).

In 2004 a study done at MIT confirmed that cancer is not a genetic disease. They took a nucleus from a cancer cell and transplanted it into a normal cell, and the result was nothing. The cell did not become a cancer cell. When they took mitochondria from a cancer cell and transplanted it into a normal cell, the result showed that the cell became a cancer cell.

Despite all the evidence, the medical world still clings to this irrelevant dogma, and any possible cure therefore, are based on an incorrect premise and can never yield a cure. I could not believe it. Surely a significant discovery such as the fact that cancer is a mitochondrial disease would steer cancer research on a new path, a path that in my view, would yield a cure.

So, I was wondering, if the basic premise of cancer is misunderstood by the medical community that treats us for cancer, what else have they missed? I intensified my study. Here are some key insights: (I have quoted some of these verbatims to ensure that I do not change the information or the context in which it is presented)

The link between fibroblasts and cancer

"Cancer is associated with fibroblasts at all stages of disease progression, including metastasis, and they are a considerable component of the general host response to tissue damage caused by cancer cells. Fibroblasts can survive conditions of extreme stress, which is lethal to all other cells." (Kalluri R, 2016).

What are fibroblasts?

Fibroblasts are the primary connective tissue cells in the body. There are two states of this cell type: firstly, fibroblasts when these cells are in an activated state. Fibrocytes when they are less active and are involved in tissue maintenance and metabolism. As we can see, the existence of fibrocytes is crucial to our bodies as it is responsible for making the extracellular matrix and collagen.

The link between oxidative stress and cancer

"Extensive research during the last two decades has revealed the mechanism by which continued oxidative stress can lead to chronic inflammation, which in turn could mediate most chronic diseases including cancer, diabetes, cardiovascular, neurological and pulmonary diseases. Indeed, cancer initiation and progression has been linked to oxidative stress by increasing DNA mutations or inducing DNA damage, genome instability, and cell proliferation." (Reuter et al., 2010).

What is oxidative stress?

"ROS (reactive oxygen species) is one of the main causes of cellular stress. The survival of a cell depends on the balance between oxidants (oxygen and ROS) and antioxidants (enzymes and proteins such as glutathione, catalase or superoxide dismutases). Normally, the cell can fight against the oxidative stress and survive, but if the oxidant-antioxidant balance is too deregulated for the cell to correct it, the cell dies. Producing ROS is a normal part of cellular respiration. This can easily be countered by superoxide dismutases, which is an enzyme that helps break down potentially harmful oxygen molecules in cells, which might prevent damage to tissues." ("Superoxide Dismutase", 2001).

Despite this evidence that cancer is so strongly linked to oxidative stress, the reduction of oxidative stress does not receive attention in cancer therapy programmes. I have only found one so far where the reduction of oxidative stress is addressed as part of the cancer treatment plan. There are many medical research articles available that point to the control of oxidative stress as a potential anticancer therapy.

The relationship between iron and cancer
"Dysregulation of the iron metabolism can increase cancer risk and promote tumour growth. Cancer cells exhibit an enhanced dependence on iron, a phenomenon called iron addiction. Work concluded in the past few years has revealed new cellular processes and mechanisms that deepen our understanding of the link between iron and cancer. Numerous laboratory and clinical investigations over the past few decades have observed that one of the dangers of iron is its ability to favour neoplastic cell growth. The metal is carcinogenic due to its catalytic effect on the formation of hydroxyl radicals, suppression of the activity of host defence cells and the promotion of cancer cell multiplication. In both animals and humans, primary neoplasms develop at body sites of excessive iron deposits. Procedures associated with lowering host iron intake and inducing host cell iron efflux can assist in the prevention and management of neoplastic diseases. Iron is an essential nutrient that facilitates cell proliferation and growth. However, iron also has the capacity to engage in redox cycling and free radical formation. Therefore, iron can contribute to both tumour initiation and tumour growth; recent work has also shown that iron has a role in the tumour microenvironment and in metastasis. Targeting iron metabolic pathways may provide new tools for cancer prognosis and therapy." (Torti et al., 2014).

"Thus, modulation of the ferroptotic and ferritinophagic processes may be potential targets for the development of novel therapeutic treatment strategies for cancer in addition to iron chelators which deplete intracellular iron essential for cancer cell survival." (Lui et al., 2015).

The role of the immune system in fighting cancer

"Our immune system does attack cancer cells," says Professor Tim Elliott, a Cancer Research UK-funded immunologist from the University of Southampton.

"Cancer immunotherapy is becoming an appealing and attractive strategy among different therapeutic options over the past years and has shown its power against malignancies. It utilizes the body's immune system to induce an anti-tumour response, and thus, cancer can be defeated. Several clinical trials have investigated their potentials in cancer patients' life savings, and after witnessing the amazing effect of cancer immunotherapy, it was selected as *2013's Breakthrough of the Year* by Science magazine." (Zhang & Chen, 2018).

After all my research, what could I conclude about cancer? At this point, what did I know about cancer that could help me? In my case, everything I needed to know.

I had enough evidence to convince me that cancer is not a genetic disease but a metabolic disease. This was confirmed when I discovered the fundamental difference between a cancer cell and a normal cell. During my study of the energy production of cells, I became greatly interested in oxidative stress and followed the link through to cancer: oxidative stress plays a role from the start to the spreading of cancer. As I delved deeper into cancer, I found the relationship between iron and cancer and the role of iron in cancer initiation and tumour growth. I also discovered that intracellular iron is essential for cancer cell survival. Lastly, I wanted to know why our immune system is not fighting cancer. As it turns out, our immune system can fight cancer.

Based on my research, I had to rectify the following in my body:
- I reduced oxidative stress.
- I regulated my iron metabolism.
- I strengthened my immune system.

At this point, I don't expect you to understand this chapter. I wrote it to show you that I based the treatment approach of my cancer on scientific research. By the time that I had finished all of my research and put the pieces of the puzzle together, I already had radiation and was busy with my 4th chemotherapy. My chance to prove my theory to myself came in December 2018 when my cancer count went from 109 to 129, and I stopped chemotherapy.

In my opinion, the higher cancer count in December was evidence that chemotherapy is now doing more harm than good. Without any further conventional cancer treatments, my counts came down to where I currently am at 41. (A CA15-3 count below 30 is normal for a healthy person). I did this amidst protests from family, friends and my medical team who all assured me that I am playing with my life. My answer to that was: "I did my research, scientific research. I know that I am right."

The recurrence of cancer

When talking about cancer coming back, it helps to define exactly what a recurrence is:

A cancer recurrence refers to cancer that returns (comes back, relapses, or recurs) after a period of time during which cancer has remission (usually meaning that there is no evidence of disease (NED) and the cancer is not detected on scans.) While there is not a precise definition of how much time that must pass during which someone is cancer-free and when cancer is considered a recurrence, oncologists believe that cancers which recur within three months are a progression rather than a recurrence.

Why does cancer come back? I was never aware of how many patients would have to deal with cancer a second time and maybe a third or fourth time. According to statistics from *Cancer Today,* one out of six people will face cancer for a second time.

After I survived cancer for the first time, I thought I had made it. I was unaware of the statistics, and no one told me what my chances were of contracting cancer for a second time. Considering these statistics, we must make sure that our cancer does not come back. Here are some things to consider:

As we have seen, oxidative stress can cause cancer to return, so make sure that you adapt your post-cancer lifestyle in such a way as to minimize oxidative stress. Here are some scholarly articles that address the role of oxidative stress in cancer reoccurrence:

Mitochondrial oxidative stress drives tumor progression and metastasis: should we use antioxidants as a key component of cancer treatment and prevention?
(https://bmcmedicine.biomedcentral.com/articles/10.1186/1741-7015-9-62)

Free radicals in chemotherapy induced cytotoxicity and oxidative stress in triple negative breast and ovarian cancers under hypoxic and normoxic conditions (https://hal.archives-ouvertes.fr/hal-01815246/document)

Oxidative Stress, Tumor Microenvironment, and Metabolic Reprogramming: A Diabolic Liaison
(https://www.hindawi.com/journals/ijcb/2012/762825/)

What I don't understand is why the websites that talk about cancer do not mention oxidative stress, yet there is an abundance of research to support this. In Chapter Three, you will find more information on dealing with oxidative stress.

Regulate your iron metabolism, here is an interesting article that highlights the role of excess iron in cancer reoccurrence, with specific reference to breast cancer.
Does iron have a role in breast cancer?
(https://www.ncbi.nlm.nih.gov/pmc/articles/PMC2577284/)

Keep your immune system healthy. As we have seen, your immune system plays a role in attacking cancer.

Regular testing as a method to monitor your post-cancer life. Test regularly. The cancer blood test is not very expensive, and I have mine tested every three months now.

For other forms of cancer, where the blood test route is not available, investigate how you can tell if the cancer is still at bay. Please look at the side effects of the tests. Some tests do cause oxidative stress. Here you must rely on your judgement. In large doses, radiation can cause severe tissue damage and increase a person's risk of developing cancer later. The low doses of radiation used for imaging tests might increase a person's cancer risk slightly, but it's important to put this risk into perspective. There is a lot of information out there, so gather your information and make an informed decision. Also, bear the cost in mind, some tests are more expensive than others.

Don't fear Cancer

Where does the fear of cancer come from? I know why I fear cancer. Everyone that I have known to have cancer in my earlier years died as a result of cancer. In my mind, cancer was a killer, and there was little to be done about it. Later, when I went through cancer myself, my oncologists used fear-based messages such as: "You can only survive this if you do exactly as I say." This only increased my fear of cancer.

Let's turn to research and see what other reasons we can uncover: Vrinten et al. (2017) had the following to say about fearing cancer:

"Cancer has long inspired fear, but the effect of fear is not well understood; it seems both to facilitate and to deter early diagnosis behaviours. Fears of cancer emanated from a core view of cancer as a vicious, unpredictable, and indestructible enemy, evoking fears about its proximity, the (lack of) strategies to keep it at bay, the personal and social implications of succumbing, and fear of dying from cancer."

If we can understand why we fear cancer, we can do something about it. Once we stop fearing cancer, we will be able to talk about it so that our understanding of cancer will grow, and we empower ourselves with knowledge. Looking at the above, a better understanding of what cancer is will change the view that "cancer is a vicious, unpredictable and indestructible enemy". If we understand exactly what cancer is, we will know how to keep it at bay, and then we will no longer fear that we will die from cancer, because we know that it is curable for the most part.

Psychological stress is a significant contributor to oxidative stress. So, by stressing about your health, if you are going to die and how will the people cope that you leave behind, not to mention the additional financial stress, you are damaging your chances of recovery by producing more oxidative stress. If you have nothing else to prove it to you, I am still here, and I made a speedy recovery from stage 4 breast cancer. Rest assured cancer is not the killer you think it is. Stop fearing cancer. Instead, talk about it and inform yourself about it.

What is needed for a successful recovery?

Deal with the diagnosis

It is said that your life can change in one second. You know how long a second is when you hear the news that you have cancer. At that very moment, my whole life stood still. It was like I was standing outside my life looking in on this bizarre scene, where the doctor is almost in tears, and you feel completely numb. The next minute you see the angel of death standing in front of you as you realise what the doctor just told you. Your world starts spinning. You think of your children and your spouse. How will they cope without you? You think of all the things you still wanted to do, and now it is too late. Life will never be the same again.

The first question that comes up in the patient's mind is, *why me?* Why did I have to get cancer? I am a good person, and I do good things. Cancer is not a whip that is used to punish evil people on earth. It is just a disease, and you can beat this. Therefore, this question is not helpful. A lot of patients get stuck with this question in their minds, and this takes valuable time away from them that they could have focused on managing their therapy properly and being positive about their healing journey.

Accept the fact that you have cancer and that it is *temporary*. You are going to make it and must decide that you want to recover from this and then take it one day at a time. You know that life will never give you a challenge without the necessary tools and skills to deal with it successfully. Use this opportunity to decide that you are going to do whatever it takes and that you *are* going to recover.

Another important thing to remember is that your diagnosis is not cast in stone. There are countless examples of people who were given three months to live. They decided to get their affairs in order, sold their businesses and divided their possessions amongst their children, only to be still living four years later.

Remember, you are not dead yet. Make plans for your future and not for your funeral. Go out and sit in the sun or under a tree, reconnect with your hobbies and your passions if you can. Use this opportunity to recover and find yourself again. Sometimes, life is so hastened that we lose ourselves along the way. Here you have a couple of months if you are not able to work, to find yourself again and reconnect with yourself.

Live fully until your last breath. It is coming, but you do not have to die from cancer. Be positive and optimistic about your future and always find something to smile about. You are so much more fortunate than many other people. You are loved and taken care of. Many people must die alone in an ally, without anyone by their side or anyone to miss them when they are gone. You are fortunate.

There are obvious cancer questions that the patients ask their oncologists:

How bad is it?
This mostly refers to the staging of cancer. Cancer is staged from one to four, with four being the most severe. You need to know what each stage represents and that it is merely a way for the doctors to determine what course of treatment is most likely to be effective. It is not a death sentence. It is important to note that cancer staging is not an exact science. Doctors are learning more about it all the time. Let's look at the staging of cancer in more detail:

Most cancers that involve a tumour are staged in five broad groups. These are usually referred to with Roman numerals. Other kinds, like blood cancers, lymphoma, and brain cancer, have their own staging systems, but they all tell you how advanced the cancer is. For more detailed information, please visit:

Stages of Cancer (https://www.webmd.com/cancer/cancer-stages#1)

Stage 0 means there's no cancer, only abnormal cells with the potential to become cancer.

Stage I means the cancer is small and only in one area.

Stage II and III mean the cancer is larger and has grown into nearby tissues or lymph nodes.

Stage IV means cancer has spread to other parts of your body. It's also called advanced or metastatic cancer.

How long will I live?

This is a complicated question and depends on so many factors that the best your oncologist can do is to estimate from similar cases from their experience. I mention this because it is so important that you do not take this as a final answer. By managing your cancer treatment properly, you will astound both yourself and your oncologist. Therefore, it is crucial to become a partner in your recovery journey and manage your therapy properly.

What will my quality of life be like?

This depends much more on you than on cancer itself. The treatment side effects can effectively be managed, like the side effects from chemotherapy, and if you have metastasis into the bones, this can also be rectified. It all depends on how much you are prepared to do. Medical aids do not cover a lot of complementary therapies, and you will need to pay for these yourself, however, if the results are positive as they were in my case, you cannot put a price on that.

I went from "we will try to get you mobile again" to walking within three months, which astounded everybody. I, therefore, determined the quality of my life and not my oncologist.

The Battle in your own mind

This is one of the most significant steps you must take on your recovery journey. You must be positive. You are going to recover; there must be no doubt in your mind about this. The best way to stay positive is to be grateful for everything that you have.

Be grateful that you are still here, that another day was added to your life. Understand this and hear me very clearly: *You do not need cancer to die*. You could also die in a car accident or from anything else. This one thing is absolutely guaranteed. You are not going to live forever. You will die, but you do not want to die from cancer.

Let something else take you from this place, but not cancer. Forget about all the people that you know that have died from cancer. You are different, and you will make it. You have this book to guide you to manage your therapy; you have the advantage.

Just listen to your body and your instincts. You are a survivor. This is where the biggest part of the cancer battle is won in your own mind. If you worry that you are not going to make it, you are only contributing to stress, and this is not helpful. Stress will only make your cancer worse; you are not dead yet; cancer is not a death sentence. Determine for yourself that you will *live*.

Do not worry about your family. They are fine. Do not worry about what will happen to them should you die; this only creates doubt in your mind that you might not make it. Be positive when you speak to people about your recovery. "The word has become flesh" which means believe it and speak healing words. You are recovering and doing very well.

Celebrate every small sign on your recovery journey; this will give you the positive attitude that you need to beat this. Avoid negative people at all costs, even if you hurt their feelings. This is about you, not about them.

You need to take your recovery seriously and do whatever you can to make it. Put yourself first, be selfish and avoid drama-seekers.

One's mind does become overwhelmed by thoughts of cancer. It is, therefore, of the utmost importance that you keep your mind busy. Learn something new or do things (that you can) for other people. During my recovery, I transcribed radio interviews, and I studied for a skincare formulator. You can do the same, keep yourself busy in a meaningful way. The more you keep yourself busy with other things, the less you are going to think about your cancer. This is of crucial importance to your recovery.

Try and stick to your routine as best you can. Get up in the mornings, even if you lie down shortly after. It doesn't matter, and the most important thing is to feel that you are still you. Despite the cancer challenge, you can still function, even if you end up in a wheelchair for a short time like I did.

In the beginning, I could not reach my feet to put cream on them, and then slowly, I was able to start reaching and eventually I rubbed my own feet with cream. To a normal person, this might sound silly, but cancer survivors thrive on all and any signs of recovery.

Become a partner in the management of your recovery

Why am I so adamant that you should assist in the management of your therapy? Here I will cite two examples and remember, I was under private care that cost a fortune. Even in state hospitals, such mistakes would not be acceptable, but I want to show you how things can go wrong.

Firstly, the very first chemotherapy that I had in 2014, was administered by a qualified oncologist who has been doing this for many years; I got my chemotherapy undiluted. Had I not left this oncologist and gone to a new one I would have never discovered this mistake.

In addition to the weight loss, I ended up with a severe chemotherapy brain, to such a degree that I could not go anywhere on my own, because I would lose my car in the parking lots. I was also so weak from the chemotherapy that I could not walk more than twenty meters without having to stop. Note that before my cancer, I was very active and in good physical shape.

The second example is the administration of Zoledronic Acid. It states explicitly that it cannot be given with other medicines, not even in the same vein as other medicines. So, I was horrified when they wanted to administer it in the same IV. The doctor just shrugged his shoulders. I could not believe this. This was when I left my first oncologist in 2018.

When I left the first oncologist that treated me in 2018, I told her that I was very unhappy with her service. She hardly spent any time explaining anything to me; she merely rattled off her diagnosis and that I will undergo radiation and chemotherapy. She told me that she has so many patients to see every day that she could not give individual attention.

I almost fainted, excuse me. I am trying to fight a life-threatening disease, and I am not getting individual attention, what was I getting then? A recipe that she has concocted for every woman presenting with stage 4 breast cancer. We as their patients deserve proper care and attention, and we must expect that medicines will be administered correctly. I suggested to her to rather see fewer patients and do a proper job. It is not like we have the flu. Cancer is one of the biggest killers in the world, and this is one of the reasons why. Please make sure that you get an oncologist that takes the time to listen, explain and give you individual attention.

I cannot stress this enough: you need to question everything until you are happy and satisfied. Make sure that you have enough information to make the right decision about your therapy. Ask your oncologist to explain your results properly. I have used my blood tests as an example in Appendix A to elucidate the importance of every part of the blood test. If it were not significant, they would not have tested for it. You need to know what the significance of every test is and, more importantly, knowing if there is progress, do the counts have to come down, for example, and what are the normal ranges for the counts.

Please do not leave your recovery in the hands of your oncologist. Become a partner in the management of your recovery journey. An oncologist is there to advise on possible treatments and prescribe them if you agree to them. A lot of oncologists will act as if you must listen to them and you must follow their advice. This is not at all necessary. They must explain your condition to you as they understand it and have interpreted it from the tests. Based on these facts, they must present you with options, and you (having been given brain cells to think with) must weigh the evidence and make your decision.

You cannot weigh the evidence thoroughly and fairly if you do not understand what your oncologist is telling you. *Ask questions*. Ask them to explain it in laymen's terms, if you were not given options, ask them to provide you with options. If they get upset with you, they do not deserve to serve you.

You have a brain; you can get information on your specific cancer, and you can assist in managing your therapy. For example, I insisted on only taking a 75% chemotherapy dosage, and I monitored my progress very closely. I made this decision because the first time I had chemotherapy, they started me on 100% dosage and I almost died within two months, ending up at 47kg.

My approach worked; the camel milk with the 75% chemotherapy was all I needed, although my oncologist was not happy that I was prescribing how much chemotherapy I will take. I was insistent.

My recovery from stage 4 breast cancer was much easier than the previous time, which was only stage 3 because I managed my therapy correctly. I educated myself by gaining a proper understanding of how cancer starts and grows as best I could from reliable medical sources. This was rather difficult as I do not have biochemistry or medical background, but through persistent study, I had enough information to work within two months of constant research.

Do not take everything your oncologist says as the gospel. If your doctor prescribes radiotherapy, ask them what the side effects will be. Go and search on the internet and see if this corresponds with what the doctor told you. If it does not, then go to them and ask them about it. Maybe you understood wrongly, or perhaps they left some information out because they do not think that you will need it.

Radiation has side effects, that is for sure, but you need to know what to expect so that you will know when something is very wrong. After my 5th radiation session, I told my oncologist that I am not happy and that I need my file to go back to my previous oncologist. She was upset, but I insisted, even when she told me that the side effects were normal. When I walked into my old oncologists' room, it took him two minutes to see that I was in severe pain. After an x-ray, it was established that my intestines were so blocked from the radiation and all the painkillers I was on. Some tummy medication sorted that out very quickly, and I returned to have my last five sessions. It is noteworthy to mention that my own oncologist and two emergency room doctors failed to diagnose this problem correctly. Every time I was treated for an ulcer, which by the way I did not have. This is to illustrate to you how important it is to manage your therapy properly. If your doctor does not want to listen to you, find another one. There are plenty of good oncologists who will see you.

You need to know what the side effects of all your medications are, even if they are painkillers. Make a list of all the side effects with the names of the medicines and how often you take them and paste it on the fridge, or some other convenient place. When you need to be rushed to the emergency room like I was, this information is very valuable to the attending doctor in the ER. It is of crucial importance that you know what specific chemotherapy you are on. All chemotherapies have different side effects. Get the pamphlet with all the side effects from your oncologist or you can also find it online. This information should also be added to your list on the fridge, in case of an emergency.

The first step in managing your therapy will be to ensure that all the relevant medical tests are done.

What tests are needed to diagnose cancer accurately?

I specifically included this section because my first oncologist did not do nearly enough tests to ensure that there is enough information to track my recovery progress accurately. Make sure you have all the relevant information to establish a proper baseline from which you can monitor your progress on your journey to recovery. During my first visit to my second oncologist, she mentioned that the tests done by the first oncologist are not sufficient to base a treatment plan on. For example, my bone density was never tested, and a lot of crucial blood tests were missing.

Here I urge you to do your research. Google for tests that are used for your type of cancer and make sure that your oncologist establishes a proper baseline through relevant tests so that you can monitor and track your progress. To help you on your research journey here are some classes of tests that are done as stated by the American Cancer Society:

- Blood tests
- Complete blood count (CBC)
- Blood Chemistry Panel
- Blood protein test
- Tumour marker test
- Circulating tumour cell test
- Imaging (Radiology) Tests
- CT scan
- MRI scan
- X-rays (standard or contrast studies)
- Bone scans (PET, MUGA, Gallium, etc.)
- Ultrasound
- Biopsies
- Endoscopy procedures

Because this area is neglected so often, I feel compelled to go over the CBC and Blood Chemistry Panel in more detail. This information will be very helpful to you in managing your therapy.

Complete blood count (CBC):

The most common lab test that you'll have done during treatment is called a complete blood count, or CBC. It measures three basic types of blood cells.

Each of these cells has a particular purpose, and cancer and cancer treatments can harm each:

Red blood cells:

RBCs carry oxygen to and carbon dioxide away from the cells in your body. When the Hgb and Hct values fall too low, it's called anaemia.

White blood cells:

WBCs fight infection. There are many types of white blood cells, and each fights infection in a unique way. The most important infection-fighting WBC is the neutrophil. The number doctors look at is called your absolute neutrophil count (ANC). A healthy person has an ANC between 2,500 and 6,000. When the ANC drops below 1,000 it is called neutropenia. Your doctor will watch your ANC closely because the risk of infection is much higher when the ANC is below 500.

Platelets:

Platelets help control bleeding. You may bruise or bleed easily when your platelet levels are low. The risk of bleeding goes up when platelet levels drop below 20,000.

Chemistry panel:

Another type of blood test looks at blood chemistry and measure the following:
- Fats (lipids)
- Proteins
- Sugar (glucose)
- Electrolytes (like potassium, magnesium, sodium, and calcium)
- Enzymes

Specific blood chemistry tests can show how well your organs are working. For instance, liver function studies tell your doctor how well your liver is working. Other tests look at how well your kidneys are working. The chemistry panel may also show other problems with body function.

Some treatments can cause changes in your body's blood chemistry, such as a drop in the amount of potassium in your blood. Your blood chemistry balance can also be changed by dehydration, which may be caused by nausea, vomiting, or diarrhoea. Your blood chemistry tests are crucial to ensure that side effects of the treatments are controlled. Some cancer treatments affect your kidneys or liver. Make sure that you know what the side effects of your specific treatment protocol are, and which tests can be used to track the impact of the treatment on your body.

Understanding your lab test results
Blood tests are done to help watch your body's response to treatment. They can show small changes before problems get serious. Keeping track of your results lets your doctor act as soon as your blood counts change to help prevent many cancer-related problems and cancer treatment side effects. Some people find it helps to ask for a copy of their lab results and have a member of their cancer care team go over the numbers with them. By getting a copy, you can also see what the normal ranges are for the lab that tested your blood and where your numbers fall within that range.

How to find normal values
Each lab has its own range for what it considers normal values for complete blood counts and chemistry panel results. What's normal for one lab might not quite be normal for another, so it's important to know what your lab's normal range is when looking at your results.

Normal ranges for some tests also vary by age and gender. As a rule, the normal ranges are printed on the lab report, next to your test results. Results that are high or low might have the letter (H) or (L) after the number or could be printed to the side or in a different column to call attention to the abnormal result.

The most important aspects of cancer tests are the following:
- You need to have copies of all your tests.
- Ask your oncologist to explain them to you in detail.

- Make sure you understand which tests will show the progression on your journey to recovery.

The first time I had chemotherapy, they only tested the white blood cell count to see if they can administer chemotherapy again. Much more than this is required to make sure that you are recovering with the treatment and that it is safe to continue with the treatment protocol. Appendix A, in the back of this book, is an example of some of the blood tests and what they represent.

Factors that influence a successful recovery

Most of these factors have been discussed throughout this book, so let us make a summary of them so that you have an easy reference:

Don't fear cancer. There is absolutely no reason to fear cancer. Not all of us make it, but if you manage your therapy properly and you listen to your body and your instincts, you will be one of the survivors. Do not let anybody (family, friends, and doctors) tell you that you are playing with your life when you insist on managing your therapy. Let your doctor explain all your results to you and regularly test to see when you are improving.

Hope. You will need a lot of hope. Hope is one of the most powerful things on earth. Find hope in people that have recovered, but if you do not know of anyone take my example.

The will to live. You need to decide without a doubt that you want to live and that you will live and stick to your belief. I was placed on palliative care in July 2018. In October 2018, I was in partial remission. I spent only two and a half months in a wheelchair. I stopped chemotherapy in December 2018 with a cancer count of 129, and in February 2019 my cancer count was only 82 and in June 2019 down again to 41. This demonstrates, amongst other things, the will to live and the results of proper therapy management.

When my oncologist placed me on palliative care, I decided that nobody puts an expiry date on me. I will survive this.

Support your body. Your body needs help. Chemotherapy and radiation as treatments will negatively impact your body and your immune system. There are mountains of evidence in accredited journals to prove this. The only reason that chemotherapy and radiation are still used is that the standard of care protocol does not allow medical practitioners the option to advise on alternative or complementary treatments. Doctors are forced to stick to the standard of care protocol and prescribe medications and treatments that are recognised as the standard treatment for a particular disease.

Both chemotherapy and radiation cause oxidative stress and it is your job to keep your oxidant-antioxidant balance at a good level. Rest is, of course, so important to recover, so rest when you feel that your body needs it. It will be easier for your body to recover then. Listen to your body and your intuition; they are there to guide you. Do not blindly follow advice from an oncologist who does not favour supporting your body with supplements. Chances are they have never had cancer, so they have no personal practical experience with cancer. They only have theoretical knowledge and what their patients tell them.

Mental health. Some of the nausea medication that you will be prescribed has depression as a side effect. The cancer diagnosis is enough to cause depression, let alone when you aggravate the situation with medications that cause depression. Only one of the four oncologists that I have had prescribed antidepressants. They see it as the work of your GP, but if you do not ask your doctor to prescribe it, chances are you are going to battle depression as well. Depression will cause you not to care about your recovery, and in severe cases, people just give up. Do yourself this favour; make sure that you can mentally cope, even if you need antidepressants for this.

Support from family and friends. You are not in this alone. Gratefully accept the support from your family and friends. Sometimes I used to think, "you have no idea what I am going through", this was, of course, the first time when I was not on antidepressants. Once my mental mood was stabilised, I openly welcomed visitors, and I was very grateful for all the support that I received from my family and my friends. This is an essential part of the recovery puzzle because you know that you are not alone. People care about you, and they all want you to recover.

A holistic approach to cancer treatment

There are many pieces in the recovery puzzle, and if you do not attend to them all, you will have half a puzzle and thus only half a recovery. Treat cancer as a wakeup call; as a warning to look after yourself and live the life you were destined to live. You need a holistic approach to your healing and your recovery. An oncologist will only look after a small part of your recovery, which is your cancer treatment. A holistic approach means to look after your whole body and your emotional wellbeing.

Body:
Here, obviously, you want to treat cancer but manage your therapy. Firstly, you need to test regularly. When I told my oncologist that I wanted to test my CA15-3 every three weeks to see what is happening to my count, she told me that I would not be able to see a difference in only three weeks. Yet when we tested every three weeks, this was the result 388; 734; 1168; 766; 594; 175; 107; 129.

This is a big difference to notice in three weeks. It showed me that in the beginning for the first nine weeks the cancer was growing and then it came down rapidly. When it started going up again to 129, my next count was six weeks later and was 82 and 41 in June 2019. Where other people fear to have their cancer counts tested, I could not wait for my next test to see how I have improved.

Do not blindly follow the advice of your oncologist. Listen to your body and your instinct (gut feel). That is what they are there for. Your body is going to need your help. When you receive radiation and/or chemotherapy, know that your body can not fight on its own. Any oncologist that tells you not to supplement your body during any of these therapies should rather not treat patients. If a particular supplement is not approved by your oncologist, ask them why. They also need to give you evidence; otherwise, use your brain cells and Google. My first oncologist, for example, said that I may not take Vitamin C while undergoing radiation. Sure enough, if you receive a lot of radiation, you cannot take Vitamin C, but I was only scheduled for 10 sessions; thus, her advice was detrimental to my health. Vitamin C is an antioxidant (by now, you know how important these are in your recovery), and it also supports your immune system. This is crucial as chemotherapy and radiation both have severely adverse effects on your immune system. You still need to support your immune system to make sure that your body can cope with the treatment.

Let's look at some beneficial supplements that you can use to support your body. If your oncologist tells you that it will negatively impact on the chemotherapy you are getting, they need to provide you with scientific studies to prove this. Many oncologists don't know so they just say no to supplements. Enhancing and building your immune system will make your road to recovery a breeze.

Camel Milk: Camel milk was such an essential part of my recovery process; therefore, I have dedicated a whole chapter in this book specifically about it. I first started taking camel milk to minimize the effects of my chemotherapy. I could not face another chemotherapy episode like I had the first time and was determined to find a solution. Camel milk not only gave me tons of energy, but I also did not present with any of the side effects of chemotherapy like patients usually do. Xeloda, the chemotherapy that I was prescribed, causes neuropathy in the hands and feet. It makes your hands and feet very dry, and if they crack, then they bleed. A lot of patients also lose their toenails and fingernails during this process. Most patients stop taking chemotherapy when the side effects become too severe, and they decide to abandon treatment. The biggest value of camel milk for cancer patients is that it binds to iron, reduces oxidative stress and boosts your immune system.

Vitamin C: Vitamin C is a powerful antioxidant that boosts your immune system. During my recovery period from cancer, I found it very valuable as I did not get infections easily (especially when I was on chemotherapy), and it also kept my immune system functioning correctly. Find a Vitamin C product that is delivered with phospholipids, which protect Vitamin C from being destroyed by your digestive juices.

GSH (Glutathione): This is the most abundant antioxidant in our bodies. I supplemented with GSH to assist my body to maintain its oxidant: antioxidant balance during my recovery. By correcting this balance, you minimise oxidative stress.

Water: Water was meant as a nutrient and to aid in hydration. Today, unfortunately, the local drinking water in South Africa and many parts around the world is not fit for human consumption. So, we are left with bottled water, but the PH of reversed osmosed water is slightly acidic. Please try and find bottled water with a PH of around 7. This will be most natural waters. Natural waters, also called mineral or spring water, are the best if you are recovering from any illness, as they are still packed with the micronutrients that nature intended. Some cancer therapies have adverse effects on the kidneys, so keeping hydrated becomes crucial. Please Google the side effects of your specific treatment or ask your oncologist to provide you with a brochure from the manufacturer of the product.

Cannabis Oil: I mainly used cannabis oil to sleep better. Most cancer patients have trouble sleeping, and your only choice is to get sleeping tablets. A recovering body needs a lot of rest and a good night's sleep. I also found that I did not retain water when using cannabis oil. My feet were always very swollen, and the cannabis oil relieved this. Apart from these benefits that I have experienced myself, research indicates how cannabis oil assists people with cancer:

- Protects your immune system.
- Stabilizes and eliminates acute or chronic pain.

- Reduces or eliminates nausea/stimulates increased appetite. (CDB-international, 2019)

These are all therapies that I used in addition to the chemotherapy and radiation prescribed by my oncologist. They are supportive therapies that will assist your body to cope with the prescribed cancer treatments from your oncologist and to help in negating the side effects from these therapies.

Emotional wellbeing:
Another piece of the recovery puzzle is your emotional wellbeing. Nobody can deny that receiving a cancer diagnosis is emotionally very stressful. The one minute you have a near-perfect life and the next minute it feels like you are fighting for your life. You need to make sure that you take care of yourself emotionally.

Meditation is a wonderful tool to help relieve stress, and I used it daily. I used guided meditations on YouTube, where you just listen and do the breathing and relaxing exercises. Apart from using meditation to relax and minimize stress, you can also use meditation to assist in your physical healing.

Here some of my favourite meditations that I used:
Cells Healing, body aches, ailments and disease
(https://www.youtube.com/watch?v=KMmk44VU-ds)
Cells Healing the Body, mindset meditation
(https://www.youtube.com/watch?v=oVqo5ncandk)
Self Healing, influencing cells
(https://www.youtube.com/watch?v=sXtysh9GzrA)
Cells Healing the Body, become you true self
(https://www.youtube.com/watch?v=PEBcIsTuKi8)

There are hundreds of these meditations on YouTube. I do my meditation before I get up in the morning and last thing at night. This made a real difference to also kept me positive. The value of keeping your mind positively occupied cannot be overstated. If you are booked off from work during your recovery, practice your hobbies or learn something new. This will do wonders in keeping your mind off the fact that you have cancer.

What can you do if you are emotionally unable to cope with the recovery process?
This is where the problems begin. Patients are defeated by the diagnosis and sometimes the prognosis. They blindly follow whatever the doctor dishes up as the gospel. Doctors have become so accustomed to not being questioned by their patients that many of them have developed a God complex and a lax attitude towards treatment. Patients that are not able to manage the recovery process need to consult a wellness coach that can guide them. If you feel overwhelmed and do not see your way clear to educate yourself and become a partner in your recovery process, at least get a wellness coach that has been through cancer to assist you. This is the only way that we are going to ensure proper medical care.

What is the role of the wellness coach in your recovery process?
Your wellness coach will assist you with information for your recovery journey. They will ensure that you follow a holistic approach to your healing, taking care of your body and supporting it while you are on therapy. They will also ensure that you take care of yourself emotionally.

Your wellness coach will be able to assist you in finding relevant information about your treatments so that you can make informed decisions about which course of action is the best for you. Wellness coaching is not the same as counselling or therapy. Wellness coaches assist you with ensuring that you have a good strong approach to healing. If possible, find a wellness coach that has been through cancer themselves. They will be in a much better position to understand what you are going through. Having been there themselves, they fully understand and appreciate what it takes to beat cancer and stay cancer-free.

Your wellness coach will take the emotional strain out of the recovery process and assist you in making positive choices on your road to recovery. They will also help you to monitor your progress on various levels and ensure that you reach your recovery goals. This is money very well spent if you are not able to navigate your own road to recovery.

The management of cancer treatment side effects

You must manage the side effects of cancer therapy and other medications that you receive. Cancer cells tend to grow fast, and chemotherapy drugs kill fast-growing cells. But because these drugs travel throughout the body, they can affect normal, healthy cells that are fast-growing, too. Damage to healthy cells causes side effects. The normal cells most likely to be damaged by chemotherapy are:

- Blood-forming cells in the bone marrow.
- Hair follicles.
- Cells in the mouth, digestive tract, and reproductive system.
- Some chemotherapy drugs can damage cells in the heart, kidneys, bladder, lungs, and nervous system.

Make sure that you know about all the side effects of your treatment.

What do you need to know about side effects?

Every person doesn't get every side effect, and some people get few if any. The severity of side effects varies greatly from person to person. Be sure to talk to your cancer care team about which side effects are most common with your chemotherapy, how long they might last, how bad they might be, and when you should call the doctor's office about them. Your doctor may give you medicines to help prevent specific side effects before they happen, for example, nausea medication. Some chemotherapy drugs cause long-term side effects, like heart or nerve damage or fertility problems.

How long do side effects last?

Many side effects go away quickly after treatment ends, but some may take months or even years to go away completely. Sometimes the side effects can last a lifetime, such as when chemotherapy causes long-term damage to the heart, lungs, kidneys, or reproductive organs. Certain types of chemotherapy sometimes cause delayed effects, such as second cancer that may show up many years later. The time it takes to get over some side effects and get your energy back varies from person to person. It depends on many factors, including your overall health and the drugs you were given.

What are the common side effects of chemotherapy?
- Fatigue.
- Hair loss.
- Easy bruising and bleeding.
- Infection.
- Anaemia (low red blood cell counts).
- Nausea and vomiting.
- Appetite changes.
- Constipation.
- Diarrhoea.
- Mouth, tongue, and throat problems such as sores and pain with swallowing.
- Nerve and muscle problems, such as numbness, tingling, and pain.
- Skin and nail changes, such as dry skin and colour change.
- Urine and bladder changes and kidney problems.
- Weight changes.
- Chemotherapy brain, which can affect concentration and focus.
- Mood changes.
- Changes in libido and sexual function.
- Fertility problems.
("Chemotherapy Side Effects", 2019).

How I dealt with my side effects
There is no need to suffer. Most of the side effects of your cancer therapy and the other medications that you take can be managed successfully. You have already made a list of all the side effects. Here is how I managed my side effects:

Camel milk: I originally got the camel milk to assist with the chemotherapy symptoms, more specifically chemotherapy brain and the tiredness. The camel milk did wonders for the fatigue, and I had just as much if not more energy when I was on chemotherapy as I did before the chemotherapy.

Because camel milk boosts your immune system, I never once got sick. With my previous chemotherapy, it was a weekly or bi-weekly occurrence. I had to stay out of shopping centres and any places that had a lot of people with my first chemotherapy. The camel milk also kept me regular, since I was taking eight Tramacet tablets a day for the pain. I would get blocked up very quickly, besides the immense discomfort and cramps that this causes, it is also very unhealthy.

I also did not experience any of the neuropathy that is a specific side effect of the chemotherapy that I took. The other specific symptom from Xeloda is extremely dry skin. It looked like a snowstorm when I took my jeans off. Consuming camel milk and putting on a good body lotion completely took care of this problem.

Bone healing: My cancer metastasized to my hip and caused a fracture. A month later, a fracture in the pelvis superior and three broken ribs landed me in a wheelchair for two months. Due to the bone healing properties in camel milk, I was walking by the end of October 2018.

Vitamin C: I took additional vitamin C for the antioxidant benefits that it offers and to support my immune system while I was on chemotherapy and for about two months after that to make sure everything returns to normal.

GSH (Glutathione): I also took GSH for its antioxidant properties, to get my oxidant-antioxidant balance back to normal. Chemotherapy and radiation cause oxidative stress (which is caused by an imbalanced oxidant-antioxidant balance in your body).

Cannabis oil: I used this to sleep better and found that it assisted greatly with my swollen feet.

Dental hygiene becomes a problem as your gums start bleeding. You can supplement with vitamin B (ask your oncologist to recommend a vitamin B that would work the best in your case) to assist with this and use a kiddie's toothbrush. Spiderman was my son's choice when I got cancer the first time and the second time, I ended up with a green dinosaur toothbrush. It is also beneficial to rinse your mouth with a bit of saltwater and stay away from any harsh mouthwashes.

How camel milk aids in the recovery from cancer

There have been so many substances that were 'hailed' to be a cancer cure. Unfortunately, many of them were promoted without any scientific evidence to support how they act on cancer. This chapter is dedicated to scientific research on camel milk and explains how camel milk works on cancer cells.

The unique properties of camel milk
Camel milk is one of the most important kinds of milk due to its nutraceutical attributes. Camel milk differs from other mammals' milk as its chemical composition is low cholesterol, low sugar, high minerals, high in vitamin C and higher protective proteins like lactoferrin, lactoperoxidase, immunoglobulins, and lysozyme, and it lacks B-lactoglobulin.

Camel milk reduces oxidative stress
As oxidative stress plays a significant role in cancer initiation and progression, this is one of the most valuable attributes of camel milk for cancer patients.

The following study evaluated the effect of camel milk consumption on oxidative stress biomarkers in autistic children; by measuring the plasma levels of glutathione, superoxide dismutase, and myeloperoxidase before and two weeks after camel milk consumption. All measured parameters exhibited a significant increase after camel milk consumption. These findings suggest that camel milk could play an essential role in decreasing oxidative stress by alteration of antioxidant enzymes and none-enzymatic antioxidant molecule levels. (Rodrigues et al., 2009).

Camel milk contains high levels of vitamins C, A, B2, and E (acidic pH) and is very rich in magnesium and zinc (Kula, J. & Tegegne, D, 2016). These vitamins are useful in reducing the oxidative stress caused by toxic agents and magnesium is essential for absorption and metabolism of vitamins, B, C and E. (Traber & Stevens, 2011).

Magnesium is essential for the biosynthesis of glutathione and prevents damage to cellular components caused by free radicals, peroxides, and heavy metals. More recently, magnesium significantly enhances the antioxidant defence (Markiewicz et al., 2011).

The protective effect of zinc has been reported against cellular toxicity due to the palliative effect on oxidative stress and apoptosis and the activation of the antioxidant system to decreased lipid peroxides. (Marreiro, et al., 2017).

Camel milk inhibits cancer growth
Lactoferrin has the ability to inhibit the proliferation of cancer cells and protects against cancer development and metastasis. (Rodrigues et al., 2009).

Lactoferrin has the ability to inhibit the proliferation of cancer cells in vitro and repair DNA damage. The main iron-binding protein of camel milk, lactoferrin, is potent for a 56% reduction of cancer growth (Habib et al., 2013).

Dr Fatin Khorshid also suggested that anti-cancer action could be both direct cell cytotoxicity and an anti-angiogenic action (cutting blood supply to the tumour cell) of camel milk lactoferrin.

Several tumours can be cured with camel milk; very active antibodies bind onto the tumours, killing the tumour cells without damaging healthy tissue. But human antibodies are too big to do this. (Levy et al., 2013). The molecules of camel milk are 10 times smaller than those found in breast milk.

The anti-tumour properties of camel milk are due to potent antimicrobial and anti-oxidative activities that help in the reduction of liver inflammation. Camel milk is also rich with nutrients that are required for healthy liver function.

Camel milk is also shown to have potential thrombolytic action, as it causes inhibition of coagulation and fibrin formation which in turn hinders the spread and growth of metastatic tumor cells (Abdelgadir et al., 2013).

Lactoferrin has the ability to inhibit the proliferation of cancer cells. Additionally, several physiological roles have been attributed to LF, namely regulation of cellular growth, and differentiation and protection against cancer development and metastasis. (Rodrigues et al., 2009).

Camel milk regulates iron metabolism

As we have established cancer is iron addicted, and iron is essential for the survival of cancer cells. The lactoferrin in camel milk binds with the iron and deprives the cancer cells of iron. (Hosam et al., 2013). Lactoferrin is also involved in the regulation of iron homeostasis. (Rodrigues et al., 2009).

Camel milk boosts the immune system

The immunoglobulins in camel milk contribute to camel milk's incredible infection-fighting. (Gader, 2016). Lactoferrin assist with the host defence against infection and inflammation. (Rodrigues et al., 2009).

Molecules with immune function in camel milk: (Dubey et al. 2016)

Name of Molecule	Function	Reference
Heavy chain antibodies (HCAb) or variable heavy antibodies (VHH) or nanobodies	Able to interact with less immune dominant parts of antigens. More tissue penetration but similar specificity. Equivalent specifity. Rapid renal clearance in humans.	Hamers-Castermanet al. (1993); Muydermans, 2013
Peptidoglycan recognition protein (PRP)	Stimulates immune response and has antimicrobial activity.	El Agamy et al., 1992
Lactoferrin	Prevents pathogenic invasion and microbial overgrowth.	El Agamy et al., 1992 Konuspayeva et al., 2006
Lactoperoxidase	Antitumor activity. Antibacterial against gram-negative bacteria like E.Coli, Salmonella and Pseudomonas. Bacteriostatic against gram-positive.	El Agamy et al., 1992
Lysozyme	Targets Gram-positive bacteria	El Agamy et al., 1992
N-acetyl-glucosamineidase (NAGase)	Antibacterial and antiviral activity	El Agamy et al., 1992 Jassim and Naji, 2001

The unique structure of camel milk molecules

Camelid antibodies have a unique structure. They possess the heavy chains but are devoid of the usual light chains. This particular feature enhances its penetration.

Camelid proteins have a very high degree of thermal stability and are resistant to acid hydrolysis.

Camel Immunoglobulins can penetrate tissues and cells that human immunoglobulins are unable to, because of their reduced size, one-tenth the size of human antibodies thus can readily pass to the milk of the lactating camel, can cross the BBB, and be readily absorbed from the gut into the general circulation. (Gader, 2016).

What are the differences between raw camel milk, pasteurized camel milk, and camel milk powder?

Which camel milk product will be the best to use? Research shows the following:

"The parameters tested were: fat, protein, ash, zinc, iron, calcium, copper, α-lactalbumin, β-lactoglobulin, vitamins A, E, B1, B2, B6, D3, C and pyridoxal. There was no significant difference between the raw and pasteurized milk samples except for α-lactalbumin and ash. β-lactoglobulin was only found in traces." (Wernery et al, 2003).

The effect of pasteurization, which can also include powder milk, if this is done with heat, can be summed up as a lower mineral content than the raw milk and a small presence of β-lactoglobulin and less α-lactalbumin which causes atopsis in tumor cells.

Camel milk and MERS – The truth

The World Health Organisation warns about MERS in raw camel milk and therefore cautions that only pasteurized camel milk must be consumed. MERS is, however, not a disease that camels naturally carry and the virus that causes Middle East Respiratory Syndrome (MERS) has been found in bats in Saudi Arabia. This suggests a potential origin for the disease, according to a new study.

Researchers tested samples from bats living about seven miles away from the home of the first person known to be infected with MERS in Saudi Arabia. A virus found in one of the bats was 100% identical to the MERS virus seen in people, the researchers said. "There have been several reports of finding MERS-like viruses in animals. None were a genetic match. In this case, we have a virus in an animal that is identical in sequence to the virus found in the first human case. Importantly, it's coming from the vicinity of that first case," stated study researcher Dr W. Ian Lipkin, director of the Centre for Infection and Immunity at Columbia University's Mailman School of Public Health.

MERS first appeared in Saudi Arabia in September 2012 and has since infected 94 people and caused 46 deaths, according to the World Health Organization. A study found that camels in Oman, a country in the Arabian Peninsula, had developed antibodies against the MERS virus. This suggests that the camels were infected in the past with the MERS virus or a very similar one, the researchers said. However, the actual virus was not found in the animals. In South Africa, for example, there is no MERS like in many other countries around the world.

Here are my favourite articles on camel milk and cancer
There are so many research articles on camel milk and cancer. Here are some of them to get you started on your research journey, with the assistance of the chapter titled "What is cancer?" you should have enough information to make an informed decision, even if you do not have any medical background.

Camel milk lactoferrin reduces the proliferation of colorectal cancer cells and exerts antioxidant and DNA damage inhibitory activities
(https://www.sciencedirect.com/science/article/pii/S0308814613003427)

Potential antioxidant bioactive peptides from camel milk proteins
(https://www.ncbi.nlm.nih.gov/pmc/articles/PMC6116331/)

Cytotoxic and antioxidant capacity of camel milk peptides: Effects of the isolated peptide on superoxide dismutase and catalase gene expression (https://www.sciencedirect.com/science/article/pii/S1021949816301703)

The current perspectives of dromedary camel stem cells research (https://www.tandfonline.com/doi/full/10.1016/j.ijvsm.2018.01.002)

In Vitro Apoptosis Triggering in the BT-474 Human Breast Cancer Cell Line by Lyophilised Camel's Milk (https://www.researchgate.net/publication/283780642_In_Vitro_Apoptosis_Triggering_in_the_BT-474_Human_Breast_Cancer_Cell_Line_by_Lyophilised_Camels_Milk)

Therapeutic potential of camel milk (https://pdfs.semanticscholar.org/22f0/8a71c2b4236a43c9dac3c462188a99ea9a18.pdf)

Review on Medicinal and Nutritional Values of Camel Milk (https://www.researchgate.net/publication/279512531_Review_on_Medicinal_and_Nutritional_Values_of_Camel_Milk)

Anticancer Activity of Camel Milk via Induction of Autophagic Death in Human Colorectal and Breast Cancer Cells (http://journal.waocp.org/article_80077_7e3e1b16ebe93b4c57f3778071e5a2d6.pdf)

Camel Milk and it's Allied Health Claims: A review. (https://www.researchgate.net/publication/305636094_Camel_Milk_and_its_Allied_Health_Claims_A_review)

Therapeutic Effect of Camel Milk and Its Exosomes on MCF7 Cells In Vitro and In Vivo (https://www.ncbi.nlm.nih.gov/pmc/articles/PMC6247558/)

Therapeutic Applications of Camel's Milk and Urine against Cancer: Current Development Efforts and Future Perspectives (omicsonline.org/open-access/therapeutic-applications-of-camels-milk-and-urine-against-cancer-current-development-efforts-and-future-perspectives-1948-5956-1000461.php?aid=89852)

How can family and friends help?

This chapter is written explicitly for friends and family members of people diagnosed with cancer. Having been through cancer twice I understand the impact that it had on my friends and family, and I would like to give you a patients' perspective of what we go through and what we have to deal with.

I hope that this information will help you in supporting your friend or family member and assist them through this difficult time. It is not something that they can do alone, and your assistance will form an integral part of their recovery process. Recovering from cancer does not have to be a horrible experience for the patient or you as their family or friend. The first step you can take is not to take anything that they say or do personally; be the bigger person and give your support 100% no matter what.

Nobody wanted to be in this situation, and I have also included a chapter for the patients on how to deal with their demons early on, right after diagnosis to make the whole recovery journey more pleasant for everybody, including you, their dear and loyal friends and family members. Remember the minute the patient gets diagnosed; they see life through entirely different eyes, appreciate that. It is only temporary.

Coping with the side effects of cancer treatment

We usually have no idea what the therapies for cancer entail. Oncologists, in general, do not tell you what all the side effects of the chemotherapy and radiation are, and it is kind of 'the less is said about it, the better'.

What are the common side effects of chemotherapy?
- Fatigue.
- Hair loss.
- Easy bruising and bleeding.
- Infection.
- Anaemia (low red blood cell counts).
- Nausea and vomiting.

- Appetite changes.
- Constipation.
- Diarrhoea.
- Mouth, tongue, and throat problems such as sores and pain with swallowing.
- Nerve and muscle problems, such as numbness, tingling, and pain.
- Skin and nail changes, such as dry skin and colour change.
- Urine and bladder changes and kidney problems.
- Weight changes.
- Chemo brain, which can affect concentration and focus.
- Mood changes.
- Changes in libido and sexual function.
- Fertility problems.
("Chemotherapy Side Effects", 2019).

Every chemotherapy has different specific side effects. Some will make your hair fall out, and others cause neuropathy in hands and feet. There are so many specific side effects that I can't include them in the scope of this book. Encourage the patient to get the name of the chemotherapy that they receive and Google the side effects.

Do your friend or family member a favour and know exactly what can be expected as side effects. If you see some of these side effects, ask them with interest about it, what they are doing to alleviate it. You will sometimes find that patients are just so tired that another little symptom does not bother them. This is where your help as a friend or family member is valuable.

Assisting the patient emotionally

Chemotherapy patients are sometimes rude and irritable on account of being tired, nauseous, or because they are depressed. It is your responsibility as their friend and family member to look out for them and to help them where you can. Chemotherapy patients usually have emotional outbursts when they feel frustrated. They can sometimes feel their body struggling, especially people that were a very active struggle to adapt to being less active or even immobilized. You need to assure them that this is only temporary, and with the correct management of the disease, they will recover and regain all their energy and mobility.

The outburst must be seen as a cry for help. Do not retaliate try to walk away if you cannot stand it and assure the patient that everything is going to be okay. The emotional outburst is usually followed by crying, and this is an opportunity to console the patient and let them know that they are loved, they are not alone and have your support.

Do not take anything that the patient says personally. It is pure frustration that they act on. When they apologise then forgive them. Don't hold on to grudges.

Dealing with depression
If your friend or family member is on chemotherapy and they are not on anti-depressants, yet you see signs of depression, please speak to them and ask them to see their general practitioner for an appropriate prescription.

Oncologists do not prescribe anti-depressants. I am not sure why, but the depression must be dealt with. If the patient has depression, they are not able to cope with what they are going through, and many just give up. A positive mindset is of crucial importance in the recovery process.

Be patient with them, but do not let them get negative or have self-pity. This is most often the first sign that there is an underlying problem with depression, which needs to be addressed.

Assist with tasks
You need to put yourself in the patient's shoes. If you had cancer and they were your friend, what would you want them to do for you? Always be glad to help. Look for opportunities where you can help and do not wait for the patient to ask. It is difficult to ask for help continually, and it lets the patient think that you do not realize what they are going through.

Understand that they do not have a lot of energy, and if they are immobilised, put yourself in their position. Try and go to the bathroom in a wheelchair and see how cumbersome some regular tasks can become if you are temporarily disabled. Always help with a smile and tell the patient that you enjoy spoiling them and doing things for them, and when they start recovering, you will also help them to start doing small manageable tasks again.

Normal conversation

I found that in both my cancer episodes people were scared to come and visit, and if they came, all they could talk about was cancer. I so wanted to have a normal conversation about normal things with ordinary people, because this let me forget about what I am going through for that time. If you have enough of those times, cancer becomes a mere inconvenience instead of the terminal illness that you cook up in your head.

You need to talk to them about their cancer and their road to recovery, but that should not be the main topic of conversation. Treat them like you would treat your other family and friends. Talk and enquire about life in general and then ask them how they are doing and feeling.

When you talk to the patient, be positive, but remain empathic. They need to know that you sympathise with them, but self-pity is not allowed.

Regular visits and interaction

If you understand that a person on chemotherapy has very low energy levels, then you can understand that sometimes they are just so tired that they cannot go somewhere with you or watch a movie with you or whatever the case may be. Do not shut them out from your normal activities.

Help them as much as you can with their activities and keep inviting them to participate in your activities. Some days are better than others. You might get a good day, and then they will gladly join you and appreciate that you have invited them.

Don't be scared to visit them. They might look a bit worse for wear, but they are still in there; the same person. It is just the body that is taking a bit of a beating at the moment. Encourage them to participate in family activities and try to pick something that they can get involved in.

Also, encourage them to spend time with their friends and do the things that they have always done. Like I said, before there are good days and bad days, on the bad days they need you more than you realise, but they are also not going to be the most pleasant people to be around. Make sure that extended family and friends visit regularly.

Assure them you are doing well
The first thing that goes through the patient's mind when they are diagnosed is: Will my family be okay?

If there are smaller children and a spouse, this becomes an overwhelming concern for the patient. You can assure the patient that you are alright and that they must focus on their recovery. The spouse, other family, and friends can also help the children to cope with the diagnosis and explain to them what is happening.

There is no use keeping them in the dark. Honesty is the best policy; they deserve to know what cancer is and how they can help the patient in their own way. Give them a role in the recovery journey and make them part of the process. This gives them something positive to do, and it also shows the patient that everyone is fine so that they can focus on their recovery.

Cheer them on
The patient is not dead. They are just sick. It is like any other illness, so get them to focus on how well they are doing. When they start doing things for themselves again, compliment them on their progress. This gives them confidence that they are getting better and that it is just a question of time before they are fully functional again. Do not let the patient speak negatively about their circumstance or their progress; keep them positive.

Remember you still have your job, school, or whatever things you do daily. For the patient, their whole world just came apart, and possibly they will stop working while recovering.

Despite being sick, doing as many normal things as you can is the best thing for the patient. It keeps their minds occupied positively. Please do not look at the patient like they are going to die. Empathy has a place, but those looks that tell the patient "I am not sure you are going to make it" is not helpful. We can look at mirrors, and we know when we look horrible. This is when we need you to encourage us and say, "Wow, you look better! How are you feeling?"

This positivity spills over to the patient and is immensely helpful to make them realise things are not as bad as they seem for the patient.

Staying Cancer-Free

There are specific reasons that we got cancer in the first place, and most of them can be attributed to our lifestyles. Excessive amounts of stress in your workplace, bad eating habits and consumption of things that cause oxidative stress. Indeed, the most significant part of staying cancer-free is to ensure that we address all the things in our lives that cause oxidative stress and make sure that we take care of ourselves and our bodies.

Your wellness coach will also be able to assist you in making decisions around what must change for you. Many of the therapies that you have undergone to get rid of cancer, actually have cancer and tumour forming as side effects. That is one of the reasons that cancer comes back. Some cancer treatments such as chemotherapy and radiation therapy may increase a person's risk of developing a different type of cancer later in life. (American Cancer Society, 2019).

Until we have changed how cancer is treated, we have to do everything we can to make sure that it does not come back. As a reminder, one out of six people will deal with cancer for a second time. Here are some tips to stay cancer-free:

Reduce oxidative stress

"Extensive research during the last two decades has revealed the mechanism by which continued oxidative stress can lead to chronic inflammation, which in turn could mediate most chronic diseases including cancer, diabetes, cardiovascular, neurological and pulmonary diseases." (Reuter et al, 2010).

The problem is that our modern lifestyle greatly influences the generation of ROS. External causes include prolonged exposure to UV, pollution, pesticides, tobacco, alcohol, an unbalanced diet, too much sport, stress, or a nutritional deficiency in one or more antioxidants. Psychological stress is one of the most significant causes of oxidative stress. This additional load of ROS becomes too much for the body to deal with and leads to a condition called oxidative stress.

There are several ways in which you can reduce oxidative stress

Camel milk reduces oxidative stress. Research suggests that camel milk could play an essential role in decreasing oxidative stress by alteration of antioxidant enzymes and none-enzymatic antioxidant molecules levels.

GSH also assists in reducing oxidative stress. One of the major mechanisms by which cells protect themselves against oxidative stress is the upregulation of a wide range of antioxidant genes. Among intracellular antioxidant molecules, reduced glutathione (GSH) is the most abundant intracellular non-protein thiol in cells. (Du et al, 2009).

Vitamin C is also a powerful antioxidant that will help to relieve oxidative stress in your body. (Pehlivan, 2017).

Dietary and lifestyle changes. There are many nutritional and lifestyle strategies we can implement to help prevent oxidative damage. Here are some ideas for you to try. You can also consult the internet for more information.

- Avoid rancid vegetable oils; steer clear of processed and packaged foods and toss out any canola, soybean, safflower, sunflower, peanut, or grapeseed oil that is not cold-pressed.
- Eat anti-inflammatory fats found in extra virgin olive oil, coconut oil, avocados, wild-caught seafood, and sprouted or lightly roasted nuts and seeds.
- Eat an antioxidant-rich, whole-foods diet. This type of diet supplies the body with the antioxidants and cofactors it needs to combat oxidative stress.
- Stop smoking.
- Try daily stress-reduction practices such as meditation, yoga, spending time in nature, and taking "technology breaks" to alleviate chronic stress, which causes oxidative stress when allowed to continue unabated.

- Reduce your environmental toxin exposure by buying organic foods as often as possible; avoid storing food in plastic containers and try to eliminate heavy metal exposure and have a look at the drinking water you consume.
- Aim for a regular sleep schedule, avoiding blue light at night, and getting plenty of sunlight during the day helps to sync circadian rhythms.
- Treat infections. Chronic infections are a significant cause of oxidative stress and must be addressed to halt the free radical cascade.
- Get regular exercise.
- Address iron overload. (Kresser, 2018).

Regulate your iron metabolism

Camel milk assists in regulating the iron metabolism in your body. "Bioactive proteins in camel milk facilitate the primary immune system towards invaded pathogenic entities. They accelerate the defence system and the development of numerous cell lines and, help in regulating the status of iron in the body." (Harmon, 2018).

Keep your immune system healthy

"The immune system plays a pivotal role in the maintenance of the integrity of an organism. Besides the protection against pathogens, it is strongly involved in cancer prevention, development, and defence." (Candeias & Gaipi, 2016).

Cancer can weaken the immune system because it can cause a drop in the number of white blood cells made in the bone marrow. Cancer treatments may weaken the immune system. Cancer treatments that are most likely to weaken the immune system are:

- Chemotherapy
- Targeted cancer drugs.
- Radiotherapy.

- High dose of steroids.
("The immune system and cancer", 2017).

How to keep your immune system healthy

Every part of your body, including your immune system, functions better when protected from environmental assaults and bolstered by healthy-living strategies such as these:
- Don't smoke.
- Eat a diet high in fruits and vegetables.
- Exercise regularly.
- Maintain a healthy weight.
- If you drink alcohol, drink only in moderation.
- Get adequate sleep.
- Take steps to avoid infection, such as washing your hands frequently and cooking meats thoroughly.
- Try to minimize stress.
("How to boost your immune system", 2018).

We can only win the war on cancer if we

Pay attention to the leading causes of cancer

By paying attention to the main causes of cancer, we are less likely to have to deal with this dreaded disease. Learning about some of the most common causes of cancer, and what we can do to lower our exposure or risk, we can adapt our lifestyles.

Smoking: Cigarette smoking causes oxidative stress by generating large amounts of free radicals and by reducing circulating antioxidant levels in the body.

Diet and Physical Activity: A sedentary lifestyle increases oxidative stress. Conversely, regular physical activity has a hermetic effect on the body; it induces the production of free radicals in the short term but increases antioxidant production over the longterm.

UV radiation: The generation of ROS (reactive oxygen species) by UV radiation can cause possible detrimental health effects.

Viruses and other infections: Oral infections with microbes, such as P. gingivalis, increase oxidative damage; this may explain why periodontitis is linked to several chronic diseases, including cardiovascular and neurodegenerative disease.

Chronic psychological stress: People are anxious about finances, politics, health, safety, relationships etc. The chronic psychological stress doesn't just reduce our quality of life; it also promotes oxidative damage through sustained activation of the HPA axis.

Environmental toxins: The environmental toxins to which we are exposed daily are a significant source of oxidative stress. For example, exposure to particulate air pollution in urban areas promotes oxidative stress by depleting antioxidant reserves.

Plastics are well known for their endocrine-disrupting effects. However, research suggests that plastics also induce oxidative stress. In the body's attempts to detoxify BPA, a ubiquitous plastic chemical, free radicals are generated via the activation of cytochrome P450 enzymes in the liver. The induction of free radicals and oxidative stress by BPA is believed to contribute significantly to the toxicity and carcinogenicity of this compound.

Pesticides and heavy metals: They also provoke oxidative stress. Exposure to organophosphate insecticides (OPs), the residues of which can be found on conventionally grown fruits and vegetables, induces oxidative stress by activating cytochrome P450 enzymes and by disturbing the cell redox system, which reduces cellular energy and makes cells unable to neutralize free radicals. Heavy metals, found in dental amalgams, air, and soil, and our water supply, induce oxidative stress by altering the activities of key antioxidant enzymes such as glutathione peroxidase, glutathione-s-transferase, superoxide dismutase, and catalase.

Circadian rhythm dysregulation. Antioxidant enzymes follow a circadian pattern of expression in the body. Research indicates that sleep restriction induces circadian rhythm disruption and increases the expression of oxidative stress markers. Blue light exposure from LED lights and technological devices also accelerates oxidative stress, especially in the cornea of the eye.

Chemicals in your home or workplace, such as asbestos and benzene, are also associated with an increased risk of cancer. ("Cancer", 2018).

Carcinogens:
What is a carcinogen?
Substances and exposures that can lead to cancer are called carcinogens. Carcinogens do not cause cancer in every case, all the time. Substances labelled as carcinogens may have different levels of cancer-causing potential. Some may cause cancer only after prolonged, high levels of exposure. The risk of developing cancer depends on many

factors, including how you are exposed to a carcinogen, the length, and intensity of the exposure.

The most widely used system for classifying carcinogens comes from the IARC. In the past 30 years, the IARC has evaluated the cancer-causing potential of more than 900 likely candidates, placing them into one of the following groups:

Group 1: Carcinogenic to humans.
Group 2A: Probably carcinogenic to humans.
Group 2B: Possibly carcinogenic to humans.
Group 3: Unclassifiable as to carcinogenicity in humans.
Group 4: Probably not carcinogenic to humans.

Known human carcinogens:
A full list of carcinogens is provided on this website: Known and Probable Human Carcinogens (https://www.cancer.org/cancer/cancer-causes/general-info/known-and-probable-human-carcinogens.html)

The common causes of cancer listed above lead to oxidative stress, dysregulated iron metabolisms and compromised immune systems.

Oxidative stress is the precursor to oxidative damage. Oxidative stress occurs when there is an imbalance between the production of free radicals and the body's ability to counteract their damaging effects through neutralization with antioxidants. Oxidative damage is the harm sustained by cells and tissues that are unable to keep up with free radical production. (Reuter et al., 2010). Oxidative stress is linked to cancer initiation and progression.

Excess Iron and problems with iron metabolism. An over-accumulation of iron in the body, a condition referred to as iron overload, is associated with the development of several chronic diseases, including diabetes and cardiovascular disease. One of the mechanisms by which iron overload promotes chronic disease is through the generation of hydroxyl free radicals, which promote oxidative stress. (Wang et al.,

2018). Cancer cells exhibit an enhanced dependence on iron (Manz et al., 2016)

Compromised Immune system. The immune system may play a much more critical role in age-related cancer risk than previously thought. (Newman, 2018).

Proper nutrition. As many as 30% of all cancer cases are linked to poor dietary habits. (Béliveau & Gingras, 2007).

Insufficient antioxidants. Antioxidants protect cell membranes, circulating lipids, cells, and tissues from oxidative damage. Antioxidant insufficiency promotes oxidative damage. It is best to obtain antioxidants from a whole-food, nutrient-dense diet rather than supplements. Studies examining the effects of antioxidant supplements indicate that they have no benefit and may even cause harm; there are several explanations for this surprising phenomenon:

- Antioxidants in foods are packaged with co-factors and enzymes that enhance their action and may be better absorbed than synthetic antioxidants.
- Other compounds in antioxidant-rich foods may play vital roles in the antioxidant effects of whole foods, producing effects that cannot be replicated with a synthetic, isolated antioxidant.
- To help increase your antioxidant levels, it is advised that you eat plenty of colourful fruits and vegetables. Grass-fed meats are also an excellent source of antioxidants, including vitamin E, glutathione, and the antioxidant enzyme superoxide dismutase.

Change the approach of modern western medicine

Where did modern medicine, as we know it today, start? The industrial revolution began in the 18th century and changed the way illnesses were treated. Scientists made discoveries and started to understand how bacteria and viruses worked. The changes in the way that people lived and worked in the 19th century in the bigger cities led to people getting sick, while they never got ill living and working in rural areas. This was mainly due to sanitation problems in big cities and the proximity of so many people to each other that caused diseases to spread like wildfire.

Louis Pasteur opened the door to medical microbiology and invented pasteurisation. By heating and cooling a liquid, he could remove the bacteria from it. The scientific community greatly opposed his theory that germs attack the body from the environment. Fortunately, he was confident enough to continue with his work, which has laid a solid foundation for modern medicine as he invented vaccines for some of the most feared diseases.

People became confident that modern medicine is the answer, and they became dependent upon modern medicine for every ailment rather than the natural remedies that they grew up with.

The disease centred approach of modern medicine
Modern medicine mostly treats symptoms. This is called a disease centric approach. The system of medicine practised by most physicians is oriented toward acute care, the diagnosis and treatment of trauma or illness that is of short duration and in need of urgent care.

Physicians apply specific prescribed treatments, such as drugs or surgery, that aim to treat the immediate problem or symptom. This leaves a considerable gap in our modern lives pertaining to medical care, where little attention is given to the prevention of disease.

The new era of modern medicine
We need a holistic approach to medicine that incorporates the whole person as a patient that will address and attempt to correct the *causes* of illnesses and assist in alleviating symptoms. Holistic medicine is gaining in popularity under the banner of functional medicine, where healing considers the whole person, including body, mind, and spirit. "Functional medicine is the future of conventional medicine. It seeks to identify and address the root causes of disease, and views the body as one

integrated system, not a collection of independent organs divided up by medical specialities." (Integrative Health Matters, 2019).

It addresses the underlying causes of disease, using a systems-oriented approach and engaging both patient and practitioner in a therapeutic partnership. It is an evolution in the practice of medicine that better addresses the healthcare needs of the 21st century.

Patient-centred care goes beyond the disease and encompasses health promotion and individual, not protocol, driven treatment plans. It uses the best of all the fields of medicine to address the cause.

Why do we need Functional Medicine?
The epidemic of chronic diseases is on the rise in our society, such as heart disease, diabetes, mental illness, cancer, and autoimmune disorders like celiac disease and rheumatoid arthritis.

Where does modern medicine fall short?
- The standard system of medicine focuses on the diagnosis and treatment of trauma and illness of short duration, such as broken bones and appendicitis. These practitioners are drug and surgery-oriented to treat immediate symptoms and issues.
- The standard acute-care approach to medicine lacks the methodology and techniques for preventing and treating complex, chronic diseases. There is no emphasis on individual and integrative tools to determine the unique genetic makeup of patients.
- Most physicians are not trained to assess the underlying causes of disease in each individual adequately. Strategies must be implemented to prevent chronic illnesses with interventions such as nutrition, diet, and exercise.
- Functional Medicine is a strategic approach designed to determine the ROOT cause of symptoms.
  To read more, please visit:
  About Functional Medicine
(https://www.lowergwyneddfunctionalmedicine.com/about-functional-medicine/)

Change the approach of oncology

Cancer is not a genetic disease

The first thing that needs to change is the dogma that cancer is a genetic disease. Cancer is *not* a genetic disease. As discussed in the book, it has been proven scientifically many times that cancer is not a genetic disease. It has been challenged and proven to be wrong; we now have to speak up and make it known. We have to let the medical world know that we can think for ourselves and make our own conclusions and that we don't merely accept what they tell us.

Here are some insightful links that provide evidence that cancer is not a genetic disease:

Is Cancer a Metabolic Disorder? (https://www.news-medical.net/health/Is-Cancer-a-Metabolic-Disorder.aspx)

Thomas Seyfried: Cancer: A Metabolic Disease With Metabolic Solutions (https://www.youtube.com/watch?v=SEE-oU8_NSU)

Where do the current cancer treatments come from?

In 1947, when Dana-Farber and Cancer Institute founder Sidney Farber, MD, set out to find a drug treatment for childhood leukaemia. Cancer treatment took two forms: surgery to cut out cancerous masses and radiation therapy to burn them out. The possibility of treating cancer with chemical drugs and chemotherapy had long intrigued physicians but was generally dismissed because any treatment capable of killing cancer cells was thought to be too toxic to patients.

That theory began to crumble in the mid-1940s when researchers at Yale School of Medicine reported that a chemical agent could produce temporary remissions in some patients with lymphoma, a cancer of certain white blood cells. It eroded further when, a few years later, Farber achieved the first remissions in childhood leukaemia with a different drug agent. Although those remissions, too, proved temporary, they were the impetus for a massive investment in research that would eventually make chemotherapy a mainstay of cancer treatment. ("Cancer Treatment: A Look at How It Has Evolved in 70 Years", 2017).

In my opinion, the way that cancer is treated currently needs to be addressed. I believe it is the treatment of cancer now that kills cancer patients. My suspicion is confirmed by the following articles that I found:

Chemotherapy warning as hundreds die from cancer-fighting drugs (https://www.telegraph.co.uk/science/2016/08/30/chemotherapy-warning-as-hundreds-die-from-cancer-fighting-drugs/)

When Chemotherapy Kills: The Inside Story .(https://www.mossreports.com/when-chemo-kills/)

The article *When Chemotherapy Kills: The Inside Story* also sheds light on why we do not know about the danger of current cancer therapies: "Critical articles appear in journals where access is limited to those willing to pay for even temporary access. Thus, to have 24 hours of access to the aforementioned article in Lancet Oncology, you are required to pay US $31.50".

This can add up if you need to see multiple articles. But doctors usually have access to articles for free through their home institutions. So, the public is at a disadvantage in getting the information it needs to make an informed decision. It is more reliant on the words of doctors and other professionals, who may have a bias in favour of conventional medicine.

If this is not a wakeup call to all of us, I don't know what would be. In essence, we are responsible for the cancer crisis of today, because we are uneducated about cancer and the treatment thereof.

In the chapter titled 'My journey with cancer,' I cited many examples of my personal experience which led me to question how cancer is treated, most of them had to do with the incompetence of medical professionals. If you think that the word incompetency is a little harsh, let me remind you that there should be no excuse for administering medication incorrectly.

A new approach to cancer treatment
Even the most vocal sceptics of the war on cancer now admit that cancer treatment today looks nothing like it did forty years ago. Complementary and alternative medicines (CAM) are also currently being evaluated for safety and success.

A new approach to cancer treatment is termed integrative therapy, which is a combination of standard medicine and CAM practices. Due to the lack of funding, CAM practices are not advancing at the same pace as standard cancer treatment, which has received $200 billion from 1970.

The functional medicine approach has many advantages over conventional western medicine's acute care approach. The question is: can the benefits be extended to the treatment of cancer?

Beatcancer.org highlights this holistic and functional medicine approach and with good reason. Where most other cancer organisations hammer on the importance of treatment, they fail to extend treatment to the whole person, and it stays a disease centred approach. Many experts now agree that it's time to take a more holistic, long-term approach to the disease, and to pay closer attention to the overall health of patients who have cancer. That is why many practitioners, including medical doctors, have embraced the rapidly expanding field of integrative oncology, which fuses the best of conventional and alternative treatments. (Weintraub, 2013).

Oncologists
In my opinion, one of the problems with oncologists is that they have not personally experienced cancer, and therefore have no concept of how harsh the cancer treatments are that they prescribe.

Here is a fantastic article of an oncologist who contracted breast cancer:

"In August 2017, during the last month of my maternity leave, I was diagnosed with breast cancer. Initially, I was plagued by memories of the young patients I had discharged home or to the hospice for end-of-life care. Thankfully they are few – but they are the ones you remember. My experience of being on the other side of the consultation desk will shape my future career, and it has helped me to understand what goes on for patients. It has been an education in patience, humility, and gratitude."

I'm an oncologist who got breast cancer. This is what I learned (https://www.theguardian.com/healthcare-network/2018/jun/07/oncologist-breast-cancer-chemotherapy)

It truly is my hope that all oncologists will read this book. I hope that you will find at least one useful piece of information that will spur you on to deliver the kind of service a cancer patient deserves. The fact that you have a degree on your wall does not make you a good doctor; it merely states that you have achieved academically, now you must perform in the working world.

It is in the application of knowledge that the value exists. Use every patient as an opportunity to hone your craft. Ask them questions, listen to their answers, and become wiser. Let your patients be your practical training ground, and always strive to use the knowledge gained to the advantage of future patients.

When is it time to find a new oncologist?
The first sign that you need another oncologist is when they are against supporting your body with supplements. Their usual excuse is that supplements will make chemotherapy less effective. This is not true in all cases. There are particular cases in which certain supplements will have a negative effect, and they are explicitly documented in scientific research. I used camel milk (one of the most potent immune boosters) while I was receiving chemotherapy (that trashes your immune system), and my results were remarkable.

Cancer and the treatment thereof is one of the most misunderstood yet most researched illnesses in the world.

The second sign is the God complex. Quite a few oncologists think that they know everything and that you, the patient, do not have a brain and that you know nothing. The most dangerous doctor is the one that thinks they know everything because their egos prevent them from considering what you are telling them and adapting treatment plans accordingly.

A doctor can only cure a patient by listening to them and then take that information together with tests that they have done and prescribe a treatment plan. How will the doctor know if something is wrong with the treatment plan? When the patients tell them, they must listen. I have never seen so many people that are unwilling to listen to their patients as oncologists.

This is from the *New York Times* – *"Decoding the God complex"*:

"The federal Agency for Healthcare Research and Quality has begun a new campaign to encourage patients to ask more pertinent questions and to prod doctors to elicit more relevant answers."

How to enhance patient-doctor communication in oncology
The use of fear-based messages. How often do doctors say something like this to patients: "It's really important for you to do this; if you don't you might ... have a stroke, go blind, lose a leg, die or (insert a scary outcome here)." There are no reliable data to answer this question, though patients report that conversations containing such direct threats are common in clinical encounters.

The more important question is: do scare tactics work? Health communication experts call these types of messages fear-based appeals. Fear appeals create an emotional reaction to some "threat" of disease, disability or death, which in turn, is thought to motivate behaviour change. Despite decades of research on the subject, there is no consensus on whether or how fear can be used effectively to motivate long-term behaviour change.

For many patients, the fifteen minutes they have with their doctor will be the fifteen most important minutes of their day. More importantly, research suggests that appeals to fear can cause harm. (Kandula & Wynia, 2015).

Oncologists may benefit from additional training to recognize negative emotions, even when displayed without intensity. Teaching cancer patients to articulate their emotional concerns better may also enhance patient-oncologist communication. (Kennifer et al., 2009).

It is of vital importance that the oncologists spend time with their patients, ask them pertinent questions and listen when the patients talk to them. Only by listening to patients can oncologists hope to learn how to serve their patients better.

This is not a one-way conversation where the oncologist speaks, and the patients have to listen. We have to establish a partnership between the oncologist and the patients, where they both take responsibility for the wellbeing of the patient. As long as oncologists are unable to understand the value of keeping our bodies healthy enough for cancer treatments, we are fighting a losing battle.

You can do your part by educating yourself about cancer and how to keep your immune system in good condition. I know that it is counterintuitive to strengthen your immune system with supplements while being on chemotherapy that trashes your immune system, but my own experience has shown that this is how quick and positive results are achieved.

Why is this taking so long?
This is an excellent question. Why are we still struggling to find a cure for cancer? Here is the answer: It is frequently stated that it takes an average of seventeen years for research evidence to reach clinical practice (Morris et al., 2011).

There is a divide between research and practice, and this divide needs to be crossed if we are to beat cancer permanently and turn the once-feared disease into something that can be treated. Just under 700 000 people die each year from the flu in the world compared to 9.6 million people that die from cancer. If we can reduce the number of cancer deaths each year to 800 000, we have won this hundred-year-old battle.

This is my personal mission, but I cannot do this on my own. Please join me and raise your voice to fight for better cancer treatment practices worldwide. Please visit www.whatcancer.co.za and subscribe to the petition. The medical world can ignore us one at a time, but they cannot ignore us when millions of us stand together.

Appendix A: Blood tests for cancer patients

I trust this information will assist you in understanding how to analyse and interpret the blood tests. Further information can be found at

The complete blood count: A guide for patients with cancer (https://uihc.org/health-topics/complete-blood-count-guide-patients-cancer)

My blood tests consisted of the following categories:
- Haematology
- Renal Screen
- Liver Function
- Thyroids
- Hormones
- Bone and Mineral
- Tumour Markers

Haematology:
These tests are used to study the blood components. The following specific tests were done:

Erythrocyte count: this is your red blood cell count. A person with a low red blood cell count may feel tired or short of breath. You must keep an eye on your red blood cell count as they can be damaged by some of the therapies that your oncologist prescribes. The good news is that this damage only lasts for a short time, but make sure that it stays within the reference range.

Haemoglobin is what gives red blood cells their colour and carries oxygen from the lungs to the tissues.

Haematocrit: measures the percentage of red blood cells in the sample of blood.

MCV: this measures the size of your red blood cells. Red blood cells larger than 100 fL are considered macrocytic. When the cells grow too large, there are fewer of them than there needs to be, and they carry less haemoglobin. This means the blood is not as oxygen rich as it should be. Low blood oxygen can cause a range of symptoms and health problems. ("MCV Mean Corpuscular Volume", 2017).

MCH levels are the average amount of haemoglobin that is in each red blood cell. This is one of the factors that can cause anaemia. (Johnson, 2017).

MCHC (A low mean corpuscular haemoglobin concentration) shows that someone's red blood cells do not have enough haemoglobin. Haemoglobin is an iron-rich protein, and a lack of it may indicate anaemia. Factors that cause low levels of haemoglobin include fewer blood cells being produced; red blood cells being destroyed faster than they can be produced; and blood loss. (Ingleson, 2017).

RDW - The red cell distribution width (RDW) blood test measures the amount of red blood cell variation in volume and size.

Platelets - Thrombocytopenia is a condition caused by a low number of platelets in the blood. Platelets are also called thrombocytes. They are made in the bone marrow and help the blood to clot. People with a low number of platelets may bleed or bruise easily, even after a minor injury. A low platelet count increases the risk of bleeding, especially from the mouth, nose and gastrointestinal tract. ("Low Platelet Count", 2019).

Leukocyte count: Neutropenia and leukopenia are terms used to refer to lowered numbers of white blood cells (WBCs) in the blood. WBCs help the body fight infection and disease. When WBC counts are low, there is a higher risk of infection.

Neutrophils count: The real number of white blood cells (WBCs) that are neutrophils. The absolute neutrophil count is commonly called the ANC.

Lymphocytes: A high white blood cell count may indicate that the immune system is working to destroy infection. It may also be a sign of physical or emotional stress. People with particular blood cancers may also have high white blood cells counts. A low white blood cell count can signal that an injury or condition is destroying cells faster than they are being made, or that the body is producing too few of them. White blood cells make up around 1% of all blood cells, and they are essential to regular function in the immune system. White blood cells are also known as leukocytes.

Monocytes are a type of white blood cell that fight certain infections and help other white blood cells to remove dead or damaged tissues, destroy cancer cells, and regulate immunity against foreign substances. Monocytes are produced in the bone marrow and then enter the blood, where they account for about 1% to 10% of the circulating white blood cells (200 to 600 monocytes per microliter of blood). After a few hours in the blood, monocytes migrate to tissues (such as spleen, liver, lungs, and bone marrow tissue), where they mature into macrophages. Macrophages are the primary scavenger cells of the immune system.

Eosinophilia is a higher than normal level of eosinophils. Eosinophils are a type of disease-fighting white blood cell. This condition most often indicates a parasitic infection, an allergic reaction or cancer. (Eosinophilia, 2018).

Basophils: Your body naturally produces several different types of white blood cells. White blood cells work to keep you healthy by fighting off viruses, bacteria, parasites, and fungi. Basophils are a type of white blood cell. Although they're produced in the bone marrow, they're found in many tissues throughout your body. They're part of your immune system and play a role in its proper function. If your basophil level is low, it may be due to a severe allergic reaction. If you develop an infection, it may take longer to heal. In some cases, having too many basophils can result from certain blood cancers.

ESR: Sed rate, or erythrocyte sedimentation rate (ESR), is a blood test that can reveal inflammatory activity in your body. A sed rate test isn't a stand-alone diagnostic tool, but it can help your doctor diagnose or monitor the progress of the inflammatory disease.

Renal Screen

S-Sodium: Patients with lung cancer can develop low sodium levels (hyponatremia) for the same reasons as other patients. These reasons can include heart failure, liver cirrhosis, the use of diuretic medications, adrenal insufficiency, hypothyroidism, or renal failure. If the sodium levels fall very low, the patient may have symptoms, including nausea/vomiting, headache, confusion, and even seizures. (Campling, 2013).

S-Potassium: Potassium is one of the most common chemical elements in our bodies, mostly existing inside our cells. Hyperkalaemia is the term for high potassium levels in your blood. Hyperkalaemia is often caused by kidney disease, but it can be caused by other illnesses and factors, such as heart disease, diabetes, cancer, and certain medications. (Fayed, 2019). Hypokalaemia is an electrolyte imbalance and is indicated by a low level of potassium in the blood.

S-Chloride: Hypochloraemia (Low Chloride) is an electrolyte imbalance and is indicated by a low level of chloride in the blood. Chloride in your blood is an important electrolyte and works to ensure that your body's metabolism is working correctly. Your kidneys control the levels of chloride in your blood. Therefore, when there is a disturbance in your blood chloride levels, it is often related to your kidneys. Hypochloraemia is a high level of chloride in the blood.

S-TOT CO2 (Bicarbonate): This test measures the amount of carbon dioxide in the liquid part of your blood, called the serum. CO_2 levels in the blood are affected by kidney and lung function. The kidneys help maintain the normal bicarbonate levels.

S-Anion GAP: This test can help determine what is causing a pH imbalance. For the body to function normally, it needs to maintain a normal pH balance or balanced levels of acid and alkali or base in the blood.

S-Urea: This test how well your kidneys are working. Some chemotherapy drugs and biological therapies can cause kidney damage. Chemotherapy causes renal dysfunction by damaging the blood vessels or structures of the kidneys.

S-Creatinine: Monitoring renal function in patients with solid tumours and hematologic malignancies is vital to the safe administration of therapeutic agents. (Aapro & Launey-Vacher, 2011).

eGFR: An accurate evaluation of the glomerular filtration rate (GFR) during oncologic treatment is pivotal and is used to manage prescriptions, particularly chemotherapy agents. (Torres da Costa e Silva et al., 2018).

Liver Function

S-Bilirubin: A bilirubin test measures the amount of bilirubin in your blood. It's used to help find the cause of health conditions like jaundice, anaemia, and liver disease. If your bilirubin levels are higher than normal, it's a sign that either your red blood cells are breaking down at an unusual rate or that your liver isn't breaking down waste properly and clearing the bilirubin from your blood.

Alkaline Phosphatase serum: Alkaline phosphatase (ALP) is an enzyme found in several tissues throughout the body. The highest concentrations of ALP are present in the cells that comprise the bone and the liver. Elevated levels of ALP in the blood are most commonly caused by liver disease or bone disorders. This test measures the level of ALP in the blood.

S-g Glutamyl Transferase: Gamma-glutamyl transferase (GGT) is an enzyme that is found in many organs throughout the body, with the highest concentrations found in the liver. GGT is elevated in the blood in most diseases that cause damage to the liver or bile ducts. Both GGT and ALP are increased in liver diseases, but only ALP will be increased with diseases affecting bone tissue.

S-Alt (GPT): The alanine aminotransferase (ALT) test is a blood test that checks for liver damage. If your liver is damaged, it will release more ALT into your blood and levels will rise.

S-AST (GOT): The aspartate aminotransferase (AST) test is a blood test that checks for liver damage.

S-Total Protein: Albumin and globulin are two types of protein in your body. The total protein test measures the total amount of albumin and globulin in your body.

S-Albumin: Proteins circulate throughout your blood to help your body maintain fluid balance. Albumin is a type of protein the liver makes. It's one of the most abundant proteins in your blood. You need a proper balance of albumin to keep fluid from leaking out of blood vessels. Albumin gives your body the proteins it needs to keep growing and repairing tissue. It also carries vital nutrients and hormones.

Bone and Mineral Markers

S-Calcium Total: Calcium is the most abundant and one of the most important minerals in the body. It is essential for cell signalling and the proper functioning of muscles, nerves, and the heart. Calcium is needed for blood clotting and is crucial for the formation, density, and maintenance of bones and teeth.

S-Magnesium: Magnesium is a mineral that is vital for energy production, muscle contraction, nerve function, and the maintenance of strong bones. Magnesium excess (hypomagnesemia) may affect calcium metabolism and exacerbate calcium deficiencies.

Tumour Markers

My tumour markers were tested every three weeks at my insistence to gauge my progress and see when I could lower my chemotherapy dosages. The following link provides a list of tumour markers for different cancers; many other websites provide this information:

Patient Guide to Tumor Markers (https://www.oncolink.org/cancer-treatment/procedures-diagnostic-tests/blood-tests-tumor-diagnostic-tests/patient-guide-to-tumor-markers)

References

Aapro, M. & Launay-Vacher, V. (2012). Importance of monitoring renal function in patients with cancer. Retrieved from https://www.ncbi.nlm.nih.gov/pubmed/21605937

About Functional Medicine - Dr. Mark Hyman. https://drhyman.com/about-2/about-functional-medicine/

About Functional Medicine | Lower Gwynedd Functional Medicine. https://www.lowergwyneddfunctionalmedicine.com/about-functional-medicine/

AL-Ayadhi, L. & Elamin, N. (2013). Camel Milk as a Potential Therapy as an Antioxidant in Autism Spectrum Disorder (ASD). Retrieved from https://www.ncbi.nlm.nih.gov/pmc/articles/PMC3773435/

Alebie G., et al. 'Therapeutic Applications of Camel's Milk and Urine against Cancer: Current Development Efforts and Future Perspectives' Journal of Cancer Science & Therapy, 9 pp.468-478.

Alkaline Phosphatase (ALP) - Lab Tests Online. https://labtestsonline.org/tests/alkaline-phosphatase-alp

American Cancer Society. (2019). Testing Biopsy and Cytology Specimens for Cancer. Retrieved from https://www.cancer.org/treatment/understanding-your-diagnosis/tests/testing-biopsy-and-cytology-specimens-for-cancer.html

Badawy A.A., et al. 'Therapeutic Effect of Camel Milk and Its Exosomes on MCF7 Cells In Vitro and In Vivo' Integrative Cancer Therapies, 2018 Dec, 17(4) pp. 1235-1246.

Basophils: Normal Range, Function, and More. https://www.healthline.com/health/basophils

Béliveau R. & Gingras D. (2007). Role of nutrition in preventing cancer. Retrieved from https://www.ncbi.nlm.nih.gov/pmc/articles/PMC2231485/

Bilirubin Test: High vs. Low Levels, Direct vs. Indirect. https://www.webmd.com/a-to-z-guides/bilirubin-test

Calcium - Lab Tests Online. https://labtestsonline.org/tests/calcium

Camel4all | Camel. https://camel4all.com/

Campling, B. (2013). Low Sodium and Lung Cancer. Retrieved from https://www.oncolink.org/frequently-asked-questions/cancers/lung/general-concerns/low-sodium-and-lung-cancer

Canadian Cancer Society. (2017) Low platelet count. Retrieved from http://www.cancer.ca/en/cancer-information/diagnosis-and-treatment/managing-side-effects/low-platelet-count/?region=on

Cancer - Symptoms and causes - Mayo Clinic. https://www.mayoclinic.org/diseases-conditions/cancer/symptoms-causes/syc-20370588

Cancer risk may increase as immune system declines. https://www.medicalnewstoday.com/articles/320827.php

Cancer Treatment: A Look at How It Has Evolved in 70 Years. (2017). Retrieved from https://blog.dana-farber.org/insight/2017/11/cancer-treatment-look-evolved-70-years/

Cancer.net. (2018). What is cancer? Retrieved from https://www.cancer.net/navigating-cancer-care/cancer-basics/what-cancer

Cancers under hypoxic and normoxic conditions. Retrieved from https://hal.archives-ouvertes.fr/hal-01815246/document

Candeias, S. & Gaipi, U. (2016). The immune system in cancer prevention, development, and therapy. Retrieved from https://www.ncbi.nlm.nih.gov/pubmed/26299661

CBD International. (2019). Cannabis Oil for Cancer Treatment. Retrieved from https://cbd-international.net/

Chemotherapy Side Effects. (2019). Retrieved from https://www.cancer.org/treatment/treatments-and-side-effects/treatment-types/chemotherapytherapy/chemotherapy-side-effects.html

Comparing Oxidative Stress Levels.docx - Comparing https://www.coursehero.com/file/41219758/Comparing-Oxidative-Stress-Levelsdocx/

Das, Chandana, et al. "Deregulated TNF-Alpha Levels Along with HPV Genotype 16 Infection Are Associated with Pathogenesis of Cervical Neoplasia in Northeast Indian Patients." Viral Immunology, vol. 31, no. 4, Mary Ann Liebert, Inc., May 2018, p. 282.

Determining if Something Is a Carcinogen - cancer.org. https://www.cancer.org/cancer/cancer-causes/general-info/determining-if-something-is-a-carcinogen.html

Dowd, M. (2011). Decoding the God Complex. Retrieved from https://www.nytimes.com/2011/09/28/opinion/dowd-decoding-the-god-complex.html

Du, Z. et al. (2009). Role of oxidative stress and intracellular glutathione in the sensitivity to apoptosis induced by a proteasome inhibitor in thyroid cancer cells. Retrieved from https://www.ncbi.nlm.nih.gov/pmc/articles/PMC2666756/

Dubey U.S., et al. 'Therapeutic potential of camel milk' Emirates Journal of Food and Agriculture, 2016. 28(3), pp. 164-176.

Elliot, T. Science Surgery: 'Why doesn't the immune system attack cancer cells?'. Retrieved from https://www.cruk.cam.ac.uk/2019/02/28/science-surgery-why-doesnt-the-immune-system-attack-cancer-cells

Eosinophilia - Mayo Clinic. https://www.mayoclinic.org/symptoms/eosinophilia/basics/definition/sym-20050752

Ethical Principles at the Foundation of JCAHO's Ethics .... http://www.ethics.va.gov/docs/net/NET_Topic_20040427_JCAHO_Standards_Ethics_Rights_Responsibilities.doc

Fayed, L. (2019). An Overview of Hyperkalemia. Retrieved from https://www.verywellhealth.com/hyperkalemia-overview-513927

Fear-based Medicine: Using Scare Tactics in the Clinical https://thehealthcareblog.com/blog/2015/05/29/fear-based-medicine-using-scare-tactics-in-the-clinical-encounter/

Fiaschi, T. & Chiarugi, P. (2012). Oxidative Stress, Tumor Microenvironment, and Metabolic Reprogramming: A Diabolic Liaison. Retrieved from https://www.hindawi.com/journals/ijcb/2012/762825/

Fluorides, Hydrogen Air Fluoride, and Fluorine. https://www.atsdr.cdc.gov/toxguides/toxguide-11.pdf

Fong, C. (2018). Free radicals in chemotherapy-induced cytotoxicity and

Foods That Fight Osteoarthritis | SparkPeople. https://www.sparkpeople.com/resource/nutrition_articles.asp?id=862

Functional Medicine — Happy + Well. https://www.happyandwellhealth.com/functional-medicine/

Gader, Abdel Galil M. Abdel, and Abdulqader A. Alhaider. "The unique medicinal properties of camel products: A review of the scientific evidence." Journal of Taibah University Medical Sciences (2016). Retrieved from https://pdfs.semanticscholar.org/72e3/0112aa74159eeca6bc98aa1cd34cf0d314e8.pdf

Gizachew, A., et al. 'Review on Medicinal and Nutritional Values of Camel Milk' Nature and Science, Vol 12(2), 2014, pp. 35-40.

Habib HM, Ibrahim WH, Schneider-Stock R, et al. Camel milk lactoferrin reduces the proliferation of colorectal cancer cells and exerts antioxidant and DNA damage inhibitory activities. Food Chem. 2013; 141:148–52. Retrieved from https://www.ncbi.nlm.nih.gov/pmc/articles/PMC6428541/

Harmon, S. (2018). Camel milk and its allied health claims: a review. Retrieved from http://docplayer.net/92643872-Camel-milk-and-its-allied-health-claims-a-review.html

Harvard Health Publishing. (2018). How to boost your immune system. Retrieved from https://www.health.harvard.edu/staying-healthy/how-to-boost-your-immune-system

Hasson S.S.A, et al., 'In Vitro Apoptosis Triggering in the BT-474 Human Breast Cancer Cell Line by Lyophilised Camel's Milk' Asian Pacific Journal of Cancer Prevention, 16(15), July 2015, pp. 6651-6661.

Hasson S.S.A, et.al., 'In Vitro Apoptosis Triggering in the BT-474 Human Breast Cancer Cell Line by Lyophilised Camel's Milk' Asian Pacific Journal of Cancer Prevention, 16(15), July 2015, pp. 6651-6661.

HbA1c explained - Type 1 Diabetes Network. http://t1dn.org.au/our-stuff/all-about-type-1-articles/hba1c-explained/

High white blood cell count: Causes, types, and other https://www.medicalnewstoday.com/articles/315133.php

Homayouni-Tabrizi, M., et al. 'Cytotoxic and antioxidant capacity of camel milk peptides: Effects of the isolated peptide on superoxide dismutase and catalase gene expression' Journal of Food and Drug Analysis, Vol 25(3), July 2017, pp.567-575.

Homayouni-Tabrizi, M., et.al. 'Cytotoxic and antioxidant capacity of camel milk peptides: Effects of the isolated peptide on superoxide dismutase and catalase gene expression' Journal of Food and Drug Analysis, Vol 25(3), July 2017, pp.567-575.

Hosam M., et al. 'Camel milk lactoferrin reduces the proliferation of colorectal cancer cells and exerts antioxidant and DNA damage inhibitory activities' Food Chemistry Vol 141, Issue 1, 1 November 2013, pp. 148-152.

How do I ... avoid carcinogens? | Society | The Guardian. https://www.theguardian.com/uk-news/2015/oct/30/cancer-carcinogens-avoid-i-die-exposure

How does the ESR Blood Test help you? - YouTube. https://www.youtube.com/watch?v=eim34gGKwx0

Huang, X. (2009). Does iron have a role in breast cancer? Retrieved from https://www.ncbi.nlm.nih.gov/pmc/articles/PMC2577284/

Hyperkalemia: Symptoms, Treatment, and More. https://www.verywellhealth.com/hyperkalemia-overview-513927

Hypochloremia (Low Chloride) - Managing Side Effects .... http://chemocare.com/chemotherapy/side-effects/hypochloremia-low-chloride.aspx

Ibrahim H.R., et al., 'Potential antioxidant bioactive peptides from camel milk proteins' Animal Nutrition, Vol 4(3), September 2018, pp. 273-280.

I'm an oncologist who got breast cancer. This is what I https://www.theguardian.com/healthcare-network/2018/jun/07/oncologist-breast-cancer-chemotherapy

Ingleson, K. (2017). What's to know about low MCHC in blood tests? Retrieved from https://www.medicalnewstoday.com/articles/319613.php

Integrative Health Matters. (2019). What is Functional Medicine? Retrieved from https://ihm.life/about-us/

Integrative Oncology: A Healthier Way to Fight Cancer .... https://experiencelife.com/article/integrative-oncology-a-healthier-way-to-fight-cancer/

Iron - Cancer - Health e Iron. https://www.healtheiron.com/iron-cancer/

Iron and cancer: more ore to be mined | Nature Reviews Cancer. https://www.nature.com/articles/nrc3495

Johnson, J. (2017). MCH levels in blood tests: What do they mean? Retrieved from https://www.medicalnewstoday.com/articles/318192.php

Kalluri, R. (2016). The biology and function of fibroblasts in cancer. Retrieved from https://www.ncbi.nlm.nih.gov/pubmed/27550820

Kandula, N. & Wynia, M. (2015). Physician Scare Tactics Often Don\'t Work. Retrieved from http://www.payersandproviders.com/node/151

Kennifer et al. (2009). NEGATIVE EMOTIONS IN CANCER CARE: DO ONCOLOGISTS' RESPONSES DEPEND ON SEVERITY AND TYPE OF EMOTION? Retrieved from https://www.ncbi.nlm.nih.gov/pmc/articles/PMC2722879/

Knapton, S. (2016). Chemotherapy warning as hundreds die from cancer-fighting drugs. Retrieved from https://www.telegraph.co.uk/science/2016/08/30/chemotherapytherapy-warning-as-hundreds-die-from-cancer-fighting-drugs/

Kresser, C. (2018). What really causes oxidative damage? Retrieved from https://kresserinstitute.com/what-really-causes-oxidative-damage/

Krishnankutty, R., et al., 'Anticancer Activity of Camel Milk via Induction of Autophagic Death in Human Colorectal and Breast Cancer Cells' Asian Pacific Journal of Cancer Prevention, Vol 19, 2018, pp. 3501-3509.

Kula, J. (2016). Medicinal Values of Camel Milk. Retrieved from https://www.peertechz.com/articles/IJVSR-2-109.php

Lactoferrin supplement - Ray Sahelian. http://raysahelian.com/lactoferrin.html

Lavin, V. (2018). I'm an oncologist who got breast cancer. This is what I learned. Retrieved from https://www.theguardian.com/healthcare-network/2018/jun/07/oncologist-breast-cancer-chemotherapytherapy

Levy A, Steiner L, Yagil R. 2013. Camel milk: disease control and dietary laws. J Health Sci. 1:48–53. Retrieved from https://www.tandfonline.com/doi/full/10.1080/09712119.2017.1357562

Low anion gap: Definition, causes, and symptoms. https://www.medicalnewstoday.com/articles/321512.php

Low MCHC in blood tests: Symptoms and causes. https://www.medicalnewstoday.com/articles/319613.php

Low platelet count - Canadian Cancer Society. https://www.cancer.ca/en/cancer-information/diagnosis-and-treatment/managing-side-effects/low-platelet-count/?region=on

Low white blood cell count - Canadian Cancer Society. http://www.cancer.ca/en/cancer-information/diagnosis-and-treatment/managing-side-effects/low-white-blood-cell-count/?region=ab

Lower Gwynedd Functional Medicine. (2019). Functional Medicine is the Future of Conventional Medicine. Retrieved from https://www.lowergwyneddfunctionalmedicine.com/about-functional-medicine/

Macrocytic anemia: Symptoms, causes, and types. https://www.medicalnewstoday.com/articles/321620.php

Markiewicz-Górka, Iwona, et al. "Influence of selenium and/or magnesium on alleviation alcohol induced oxidative stress in rats, normalization function of liver and changes in serum lipid parameters." Human & experimental toxicology (2011): 0960327111401049. Retrieved from https://pdfs.semanticscholar.org/72e3/0112aa74159eeca6bc98aa1cd34cf0d314e8.pdf

Marreiro, D. et al. (2017). Zinc and Oxidative Stress: Current Mechanisms. Retrieved from https://www.ncbi.nlm.nih.gov/pmc/articles/PMC5488004/

Mayo Clinic. (2018). Eosinophilia. Retrieved from https://www.mayoclinic.org/symptoms/eosinophilia/basics/definition/sym-20050752

Mckenzie, S. (2019). Is Cancer a Metabolic Disorder? Retrieved from https://www.news-medical.net/news/20180807/Study-suggests-cancer-to-be-a-metabolic-disorder-rather-than-genetic-disease.aspx

MCV (Mean Corpuscular Volume). (2017). Retrieved from https://medlineplus.gov/lab-tests/mcv-mean-corpuscular-volume/

Medical Treatments that Might Affect Cancer Risk. https://www.cancer.org/cancer/cancer-causes/medical-treatments.html

Medicinal Values of Camel Milk - peertechz.com. https://www.peertechz.com/articles/IJVSR-2-109.php

Meditations by Rasa. (2016). Self Healing | Influencing Cells | Guided Meditation. Retrieved from https://www.youtube.com/watch?v=sXtysh9GzrA

Mind Set. (2015). Cells healing the body - Guided meditation (new) – MindSet Hypnotherapy. Retrieved from https://www.youtube.com/watch?v=oVqo5ncandk

Mind Set. (2017). Cells healing the body - Become your true self - Guided meditation. Retrieved from https://www.youtube.com/watch?v=PEBcIsTuKi8

Mind Set. (2017). Cells healing the body – new guided meditation. Retrieved from https://www.youtube.com/watch?v=KMmk44VU-ds

Monocyte Disorders - Merck Manuals Consumer Version. https://www.merckmanuals.com/home/blood-disorders/white-blood-cell-disorders/monocyte-disorders

Morris, Z., Wooding, S. & Grant, J. (2011). The answer is 17 years, what is the question: understanding time lags in translational research. Retrieved from https://www.ncbi.nlm.nih.gov/pmc/articles/PMC3241518/

Moss, RW. (2019). When Chemotherapy Kills: The Inside Story. Retrieved from https://www.mossreports.com/when-chemotherapy-kills/

Negative emotions in cancer care: do oncologists https://scholars.duke.edu/display/pub720505

Newman, T. (2018). Cancer risk may increase as the immune system declines. Retrieved from https://www.medicalnewstoday.com/articles/320827.php

OncoLink. (2018). Preventing Dehydration During Cancer Treatment. Retrieved from https://www.oncolink.org/support/side-effects/gastrointestinal-side-effects/diarrhea/preventing-dehydration-during-cancer-treatment oxidative stress in triple-negative breast and ovarian

Origin of MERS Virus Found in Bats | Live Science. https://www.livescience.com/39056-origin-of-mers-virus-found-in-bats.html

Part 1: The different types of cellular stress in aging .... http://www.longlonglife.org/en/transhumanism-longevity/aging/cellular-stress-and-aging/the-different-types-of-cellular-stress-in-aging/

Pehlivan, F. (2017). Vitamin C: An Antioxidant Agent. Retrieved from https://www.intechopen.com/books/vitamin-c/vitamin-c-an-antioxidant-agent

Reading Your Lab Test Results - Health Beauty Market. https://markethealthbeauty.com/your-lab-test-results/

Retrieved from https://www.cancer.org/cancer/cancer-causes/general-info/known-and-probable-human-carcinogens.html

Reuter et al. (2010). Oxidative stress, inflammation, and cancer: How are they linked? Retrieved from https://www.ncbi.nlm.nih.gov/pmc/articles/PMC2990475/

Review Current status and future directions of cancer http://www.jcancer.org/v09p1773.pdf

Rockfield et al. (2018). Iron Overload and Altered Iron Metabolism in Ovarian Cancer. Retrieved from https://www.ncbi.nlm.nih.gov/pmc/articles/PMC5545069/

Rodrigues et al. (2009). Lactoferrin and Cancer Disease Prevention. Retrieved from https://www.researchgate.net/publication/23674267_Lactoferrin_and_Cancer_Disease_Prevention

Saadeldin, I.M., et al., 'The current perspectives of dromedary camel stem cells research' International Journal of Veterinary Science and Medicine, Vol 6, September 2018, pp. S27-S30.

Sakandar, H., et al. (2018). 'Camel Milk and it's Allied Health Claims: A review.' Progress in Nutrition. Vol 20, pp. 15-29.

Serum Albumin Test: Purpose, Procedure, and Results. https://www.healthline.com/health/albumin-serum

Side Effects of Cancer Treatment - Arizona Center for .... https://arizonaccc.com/treatments/cancer-treatments/side-effects/

Sotgia, F., Martinez-Outschoorn, U. & Lisanti, M. (2011). Mitochondrial oxidative stress drives tumour progression and metastasis: should we use antioxidants as a key component of cancer treatment and prevention? Retrieved from https://bmcmedicine.biomedcentral.com/articles/10.1186/1741-7015-9-62

Superoxide Dismutase. (2001). Retrieved from https://www.webmd.com/vitamins/ai/ingredientmono-507/superoxide-dismutase

Superoxide Dismutase: Health Benefits, Uses, Side Effects .... https://www.rxlist.com/superoxide_dismutase/supplements.htm

The American Cancer Society medical and editorial content team. (2019). Known and Probable Human Carcinogens.

The immune system and cancer. (2017). Retrieved from https://www.cancerresearchuk.org/about-cancer/what-is-cancer/body-systems-and-cancer/the-immune-system-and-cancer

The Stages of Cancer According to the TNM System. https://www.webmd.com/cancer/cancer-stages

TheIHMC. (2015). Thomas Seyfried: Cancer: A Metabolic Disease With Metabolic Solutions. Retrieved from https://www.youtube.com/watch?v=SEE-oU8_NSU

Therapeutic potential of Camel Milk - ScopeMed.org .... http://www.scopemed.org/?mno=185219

Torres da Costa e Silva, V., Costalonga, EC., Coelho, F., Caires, RA., Burdmann, EA. (2018). Assessment of Kidney Function in Patients with Cancer. Retrieved from https://www.ackdjournal.org/article/S1548-5595(17)30187-8/pdf

Torti, S. & Torti, F. (2013). Iron and cancer: more ore to be mined. Retrieved from https://www.ncbi.nlm.nih.gov/pmc/articles/PMC4036554/

Total Protein Test: Purpose, Procedure & Results. https://www.healthline.com/health/total-protein

Traber, MG. & Stevens, SJ. (2011) Vitamins C and E: Beneficial effects from a mechanistic perspective. Retrieved from https://www.ncbi.nlm.nih.gov/pubmed/21664268

Understanding Radiation Risk from Imaging Tests. https://www.cancer.org/treatment/understanding-your-diagnosis/tests/understanding-radiation-risk-from-imaging-tests.html

Understanding Your Lab Test Results - American Cancer Society. https://www.cancer.org/treatment/understanding-your-diagnosis/tests/understanding-your-lab-test-results.html

Vitamin B supplements and recurrent pca - Prostate Cancer. https://www.healingwell.com/community/default.aspx?f=35&m=3999891

Vrinten, C. et al. (2017). What do people fear about cancer? A systematic review and meta-synthesis of cancer fears in the general population. Retrieved from https://www.ncbi.nlm.nih.gov/pmc/articles/PMC5573953/

Wang, Y. et al. (2018). Iron Metabolism in Cancer. Retrieved from https://www.ncbi.nlm.nih.gov/pmc/articles/PMC6337236/

Weintraub, P. (2013). Integrative Oncology: A Healthier Way to Fight Cancer. Retrieved from https://experiencelife.com/article/integrative-oncology-a-healthier-way-to-fight-cancer/

Wernery, U. (2003). The effect of heat treatment on some camel milk constituents. Preliminary report. Retrieved from https://www.researchgate.net/publication/289964575_The_effect_of_heat_treatment_on_some_camel_milk_constituents_Preliminary_report

What are Fibroblasts? - news-medical.net. https://www.news-medical.net/health/What-are-Fibroblasts.aspx

What are symptoms of high chloride? | AnswersDrive. https://answersdrive.com/what-are-symptoms-of-high-chloride-2347517

What do bilirubin levels mean? - WebMD. https://www.webmd.com/a-to-z-guides/qa/what-do-bilirubin-levels-mean

What do people fear about cancer? A systematic review and .... https://www.thelancet.com/journals/lancet/article/PIIS0140-6736(14)62138-3/fulltext

What is the normal percentage of neutrophils? | AnswersDrive. https://answersdrive.com/what-is-the-normal-percentage-of-neutrophils-2660968

What Really Causes Oxidative Damage? - kresserinstitute.com. https://kresserinstitute.com/what-really-causes-oxidative-damage/

When Chemo Kills: The Inside Story • Moss Reports. https://www.mossreports.com/when-chemo-kills/

Why Do Some Cancers Come Back? - verywellhealth.com. https://www.verywellhealth.com/why-do-some-cancers-come-back-2248952

Why is an alanine aminotransferase test important? - WebMD. https://www.webmd.com/a-to-z-guides/qa/why-is-an-alanine-aminotransferase-test-important

World Health Organization. (2018). Latest global cancer data. Retrieved from https://www.who.int/cancer/PRGlobocanFinal.pdf

Zhang, H. & Chen, J. (2018). Current status and future directions of cancer immunotherapy. Retrieved from https://www.ncbi.nlm.nih.gov/pmc/articles/PMC5968765/

"Where can I find a medical disclaimer template for the .... https://writersweekly.com/ask-the-expert/medical-disclaimer-template

www.ingramcontent.com/pod-product-compliance
Lightning Source LLC
Chambersburg PA
CBHW070659220526
45466CB00001B/499